What Stress Can Do

Why you must recognize all of the damage stress
is causing in your life and *do something about it*
by Harry L. Campbell, BPS, BCB

To Noor

Good to meet you at NYSPA

6/3/17

Harry L Campbell

ISBN: 0615981577

ISBN 13: 978-0615981574

Library of Congress Control Number: 2014905115

LCCN Imprint Name: Biofeedback Resources International, Ossining, NY

Contents

Acknowledgments

God, who has blessed me from the day I was born and gives me the ability, gifts, courage, and help to do all things.

Mom and Dad, Alfred Campbell, Sr., and Dorcas Campbell, for providing a Godly, healthy, stable environment to grow up in and an example of how to fear and love God, how to be a good person, what a normal family looks like, how to live in peace, and how to live well without being financially rich.

My wife Sophier, for not thinking I was crazy to work in a man's basement for over twenty years so that I could do something I loved and believed in.

My children, Daria and Jarrell—the best nurse and accountant I know—thank you for letting me be your hero at least for a while. Thank you for listening to me most of the time and for making me very proud to be your father.

My sisters, Ethlin and Beryl, for being my big sisters and two of the nicest ladies I know. Thank you for your encouragement, help, and being my friends.

I would like to thank my brother Freddy for being my big brother and friend. Thank you for being proud of me.

Thanks to Adam Crane for introducing me to the world of biofeedback and stress management and teaching me for so many years. Thank you for introducing me to so many interesting people, including scientists, researchers, programmers, doctors, lawyers, authors, professors, and people who spend their lives improving the lives of others.

Dr. Rafael De la Cruz, thank you for giving me my first clinical biofeedback job when I didn't see what I had already become.

Richard Zalfass, who is no longer with us, thank you for encouraging me to stop just working with the biofeedback equipment but to start to use it to help people improve their health. I'm glad that you were able to see me do it and to be around until I was able to buy Biofeedback Resources International from Adam Crane.

Thank you to those who previewed the manuscript and gave me input that helped me to improve it.

I would also like to thank everyone who has been on my team over the years who I haven't mentioned—my family, church family, friends, and loyal customers.

Introduction

What Stress Can Do is intended to bring to the attention of as many people as possible the various powerful negative effects that stress can have. It is also intended to make people aware of the fact that we can learn how to control our reactions to stress so that we minimize the negative effects. This is a simple principle, but it can mean the difference between a good or bad quality of life, good health or sickness, happiness or sadness, or even life or death.

The results of a 2013 online survey conducted by *The Huffington Post* show that 91 percent of people felt stressed by something during the month of March, while 77 percent of people reported feeling stressed "regularly," defined as at least weekly. Men and women reported being stressed equally, although the stress can be triggered by different things. More than one thousand Americans of at least eighteen years of age were surveyed.

A survey conducted by *Prevention* magazine in 1996 concluded that about 75 percent of the respondents report a level of "great stress" one day per week. Thirty-three percent said they felt great stress at least two times per week. When this survey was done in 1983, only 55 percent said they had great stress every week.

Adults report their jobs as the leading source of their stress. Stress levels have also risen for children, teenagers, college students, and the elderly. Some of the sources of stress for them include increased crime, violence, and other threats to personal safety; harmful peer pressure that leads to drug and alcohol abuse and other bad habits; social isolation and loneliness; the disintegration of family and religious life; and the loss of other sources of social support that could help reduce the negative effects of stress.

Stress in today's world is more of a problem because it is more inescapable, almost constant, and subtle because it comes mostly from threats that are more mental than physical. The stress triggers inbuilt and immediate reactions that we normally have very little control over. These reactions were originally meant to be useful in responding to physical threats.

Here is a list of some of the stress reactions and the benefits:

- Heart rate and blood pressure rise to increase the flow of blood to the brain to improve decision making

- Blood sugar rises to provide more fuel for energy as the result of the breakdown of glycogen, fat, and protein stores

- Blood is redistributed away from the stomach area, where it is not needed for digestion, to the bigger muscles of the arms and legs to allow for more strength in fighting or greater speed in running away from danger

- Clotting occurs more quickly to prevent blood loss from cuts or internal bleeding that might happen during a fight, accident, or other physical threat

Although these body reactions to danger would be helpful, even lifesaving in the presence of physical danger, they can be harmful if the perceived danger is simply emotional or mental. The problem is that the body's stress reaction is the same whether the source of the stress is a person physically assaulting you, disagreements at work with a customer or supervisor, or being caught in rush hour traffic.

When this type of fight-or-flight stress reaction happens over and over, it can lead to muscle tension, neck and back pain, heart disease including attacks, high blood pressure, strokes, diabetes, ulcers, and other stress-related sicknesses that seem to have come with modern civilization and lifestyles.

Unmanaged long-term stress can make you feel tired even after an average night of sleep, can make things that used to be enjoyable no longer enjoyable, can cause you to become unorganized, and can cause you to put off doing important things. It can make you irritable so that even small things can make you overly upset. It can make you no fun to be around. If this describes you, then pay careful attention. Your awareness of the consequences of stress should motivate you to do something about it.

Chapter 1

What Is Stress?

Sources of Stress

When most people talk about stress, they mean something bad or negative that happens that is emotionally upsetting.

Here are some technical definitions of the word *stress*:

Dictionary.com Unabridged (version 1.1):

The physical pressure, pull, or other force exerted on one thing by another; strain.

The action on a body of any system of balanced forces whereby strain or deformation results.

A load, force, or system of forces producing a strain.

The internal resistance or reaction of an elastic body to the external forces applied to it.

Physiology—a specific response by the body to a stimulus, as fear or pain, that disturbs or interferes with the normal physiological equilibrium of an organism.

Physical, mental, or emotional strain or tension: *Worry over his job and his wife's health put him under a great stress.*

A situation, occurrence, or factor causing this: *The stress of being trapped in the elevator gave him a pounding headache.*

To subject to stress or strain.

Synonyms: anxiety, burden, pressure, worry.

American Heritage Dictionary:

1.

   a. An applied force or system of forces that tends to strain or deform a body.

   b. A mentally or emotionally disruptive or upsetting condition occurring in response to adverse external influences and capable of affecting physical health, usually characterized by increased heart rate, a rise in blood pressure, muscular tension, irritability, and depression.

   c. A stimulus or circumstance causing such a condition.

2.

   a. An applied force or system of forces that tends to strain or deform a body.

   b. The internal resistance of a body to such an applied force or system of forces.

3.

   a. A mentally or emotionally disruptive or upsetting condition occurring in response to adverse external influences and capable of affecting physical health, usually characterized by increased heart rate, a rise in blood pressure, muscular tension, irritability, and depression. A state of extreme difficulty, pressure, or strain: "He presided over the economy during the period of its greatest stress and danger" (Robert J. Samuelson).

It is normal for the stress response to be activated once in a while. This is usually followed by a natural recovery or ideally a relaxation response. When the stress response is activated too often, the internal balance of the body is disrupted. If this continues too long, the body adapts so that the state of stress response/reaction begins to seem "normal." This is because the autonomic nervous system becomes retrained. The autonomic nervous system is the part of the nervous system that controls the involuntary functions of the blood vessels, heart, smooth muscles, and glands. The autonomic system is made up of the sympathetic and parasympathetic branches. The sympathetic branch tends to cause more activity, like speeding the heartbeat, and the parasympathetic tends to cause less activity, like slowing the heartbeat down. The endocrine system is a body control system made up of a group of glands that maintain stability inside the body by producing hormones (substances that cause changes within the body, like increased energy and alertness). The endocrine system includes the pituitary gland, thyroid gland, parathyroid glands, adrenal gland, pancreas, ovaries, and testes. The thymus gland, pineal gland, and kidneys (urinary system) are also sometimes considered endocrine organs. All of these systems are retrained when a person is under constant stress with no recovery or relaxation break. This can cause many mental and physical stress-related symptoms.

Change of any kind is usually at least somewhat stressful, or emotionally upsetting. This is one reason that many people tend to stay in negative situations rather than change to a likely better situation. Some of these negative situations include jobs, homes, and relationships. Changing any of these might improve our situation, but we are afraid of leaving the one we know to go to what we don't know.

In our society people are motivated to work harder and faster to get more done in less time. People who seem to like to live this way are referred to by cardiologists Friedman and Rosenman and others as "type A" personalities. They are usually in a rush, they are very competitive, and they get upset easily when they run into problems. Although many type A people are very successful, many more of them have cardiovascular disease than type B personalities. Type B people are not always worried about things being done on time. Both personality types can be successful, but type A people who are successful often pay a higher price because they are not as healthy and happy as others. Some people are just less affected by stress. These people tend to be sick less and miss fewer workdays. They don't see problems in the same way as others do. They see them as challenges instead of threats. They believe that they can deal with the situations they find themselves in. They usually also have good home, family, and work situations. These opportunities to have positive interactions with other people help them feel less affected by stress. When these same people also have healthy diets, have good support systems, and get regular exercise, they tend to get sick even less often.

Positive stress is known as eustress.

Some kinds of stress can be good, like the rush that a person gets from skiing, surfing, or other sports, or other desirable mental or physical challenges. These usually don't last very long, so the body is able to go back to its normal state shortly after the activity is over. Because these are fun and desirable activities, the body does not interpret them the same way as it would a negative stress source.

Questions

Why are we so stressed out?

Society and civilization have changed. Life moves at a much faster pace than in the past. We don't get enough exercise. Much of the food we eat is processed and includes preservatives and excess fat, and salt. The work that most of us do is not physical enough to burn up the pent-up energy that stress generates. We are bombarded with more information than we can easily process through various media. We are expected to get more and more done in less and less time. Technology has become more complex to use. Our society is in more debt than ever. Many people are unhappy with their political leaders. They are frustrated with trying to make political changes. Sometimes people don't get the desired results when they do vote to make changes. People are having more and more difficulty raising their children. Children are upset with their parents because they feel that they are overprotective. Advances in technology now allow us to receive more information than ever before, faster than ever before. We can almost instantly hear about any problem happening anywhere in the world. We get blow-by-blow, minute-by-minute updates about wars, natural disasters, terrorist acts, and anything else by television, radio, the Internet, cell phones, smartphones, and tablets. This overabundance of information can be overwhelming.

Financial pressures are increasing for the middle class and the poor. Gas prices are rising. The home foreclosure rate is increasing. Many people are losing the homes that they worked so hard to acquire. Some who are not losing their homes are under great pressure to do everything they can to keep them.

Children don't get to go outside and play as much as they used to. They don't get as much physical activity. Parents are concerned about kidnappers and child molesters. Children now have schedules. They have sports practices and games, tutoring, playdates, birthday parties, after-school club activities, and more to do. They are also evaluated on school performance more than ever.

Why aren't we doing more about stress?

I don't believe that the average person appreciates how serious the stress problem is. Many people who do know how serious the stress problem is don't believe there is anything they can do about it.

Why don't doctors tell us more about stress?

As surprising as it may sound, most doctors don't really know as much about stress as you would expect. Many doctors are suffering from stress-related disorders themselves. Many work too many hours, don't sleep enough, don't eat properly, smoke, and drink more alcohol than they should, abuse prescription and/or nonprescription drugs, and/or are overweight. There is very little on stress in the curriculum of most medical schools. It is not considered necessary for those aspiring to become doctors to learn much about stress management, stress as a cause of illness, biofeedback, or the importance of relaxation training. This doesn't make much sense to me since it has been reported that as much as 90 percent of all illnesses/doctor visits have some relation to stress, according to the Centers for Disease Control and Prevention.

I don't like to get into conspiracy theories, but there may also be a financial reason. Drug companies influence medical education, and doctors are taught to prescribe drugs. If doctors used stress management with their patients, it could greatly affect the amount of doctor visits, medication, and other medical interventions patients need. This could have an undesired financial effect on the medical field as it now exists. The long-term effect should be positive for society as a whole and for individual citizens.

What happens in your body when you experience stress?

Now let's talk about some of the effects stress can have on you.

You tense your muscles unnecessarily, hold your breath or breathe too fast and shallow, your heart beats faster, you start to sweat more, and your hands get cold. Muscles: You wrinkle your forehead, grit your teeth, raise your shoulders, clench your fists, curl your toes, tighten your leg or buttock muscles, and tap your fingers.

Chemical changes occur in the body as a result of stress. The sympathetic part of the autonomic nervous system causes some negative chemical reactions.

The stress hormone cortisol is one of the most harmful substances produced in reaction to prolonged stress. Here are some of the effects:

- Triggers buildup of fat, especially in the midsection

- Inability to relax, even when in a relaxing situation

- Difficulty sleeping

- Decrease in bone mass

- Decrease in immune system function

- Impairment of memory and learning

- Damage to brain cells

Stress also can cause a reduction in dehydroepiandrosterone (DHEA), the antiaging hormone.

Have you ever seen a person who looked older than they really were? What about a person who looks much younger than they are? Much of this can be due to differences in the amount of DHEA due to how the person manages his or her stress reactions.

Continued stress reaction can decrease production of DHEA. The production of DHEA can increase if the relaxation response is induced regularly.

The body's reaction to physical and mental stressors can cause stress-related symptoms like muscle tension, headaches, stomach upset, and anxiety.

The brain interprets changes in your surroundings and body and decides when to turn on the "emergency response." How you interpret and label experiences can serve to relax or stress you.

Richard Lazarus said that stress begins with your appraisal of a situation—how dangerous or difficult you believe the situation is and what resources you have to help you cope with it. Anxious, stressed people usually appraise a situation as dangerous, difficult, or painful, and they don't tend to have the resources to cope with the situation.

The first person to describe the fight-or-flight response was Walter B. Cannon, a Harvard physiologist. During the fight-or-flight response, a series of biochemical changes occur that are intended to prepare you to deal with threats or danger. Ancient man needed this type of response more often to react to things like wild animals. We hardly need this quick burst of energy to fight or flee in our modern society.

Hans Selye, the first major researcher on stress, found that during the fight-or-flight response, a real or imagined problem can cause the cerebral cortex, the thinking part of the brain, to send an alarm signal to the hypothalamus (the main switch for the stress response, located in the midbrain). The hypothalamus causes the sympathetic nervous system to make a series of changes in your body. Heart rate, breathing rate, muscle tension, metabolism, and blood pressure all increase. Hands and feet get cold as blood is directed away from them and your digestive system into larger muscles that could help you fight or run. You may feel the sensation of butterflies in your stomach. The diaphragm and anus tighten. The pupils dilate to improve vision, and hearing becomes clearer. If these reactions continue too long and nothing is done to stop them, long-term problems can result. Adrenal glands secrete corticoids (adrenaline, epinephrine, and norepinephrine), which slow digestion, reproduction, growth, and tissue repair and the effectiveness of your immune and inflammatory systems. When these effects are continued, the result can lead to illness.

It is not my intent to be exhaustive on the science of stress in this book. I strongly suggest that you refer to the work of Robert Sapolsky for much more detail. His book *Why Zebras Don't Get Ulcers* is a must read. I also suggest his National Geographic Special film, *Stress, Portrait of a Killer DVD*, and *Stress and Your Body* of The Great Courses DVD series. These go into much more scientific detail than I can do here.

Chapter 2

My Personal Experience with Stress

I thought I knew what stress was before. I have realized that I only knew intellectually. Book learning is not at all the same as experiential learning. I have to say that I would probably rather not know as much about stress as I do now through personal experience.

I am not trying to say that my life has been one of the most stressful ever. But for me it has been more than I felt that I could deal with at times. Things were going quite well for me in my life. I was happily married. I had two lovely young children. I had a job that I loved. Both of my parents were alive and healthy. I had a happy, healthy spiritual life and church community. I had a good number of friends whom I spent time with regularly. I laughed a lot. I considered myself a happy person. It is interesting that it doesn't matter how much you know about stress. You can't avoid it altogether. You can try to, but it finds you. It comes to you and presents itself. The question then becomes how you deal with it. Does it consume you? Does it destroy you? Does it make you sick? Does it kill you?

Things were going great for me, and then stress came. Of course I had the everyday kinds of stress that everybody deals with but nothing I couldn't handle. After all, my biofeedback business dealt with stress management at its core. I'm not sure which came first, but once it started, it seemed to snowball. There didn't seem to be much of a break. I hadn't had much time to recover from one problem before the next one started.

- Financial problems

- Being at risk of losing my house

- Marital problems

- Church problems

- Sickness of my father

- Death of my father

- A family member becoming drug dependent and going to jail

- Marital problems of others in my family

When I was younger, my blood pressure was always good, relatively low—about 110/65 to 120/70. My weight was also good—160 to 178 pounds. I was also able to lose 5 pounds in one week without any problem. All I had to do was cut back a little bit on my food intake and maybe increase my exercise a little. Life was good. I didn't really have any major stress in my life. Everything was good at work. Everything was going well in my family life. Everything was going well in my spiritual life. I could eat whatever I wanted.

I'm not sure exactly when, but probably when I was around age thirty-six, things started to gradually change. A few years later it began accelerating. I used to get exercise by walking more and driving less and playing basketball for fun. I also spent a lot of time with other people, casual friends, doing things—going to movies, playing baseball, having parties, playing cards, playing board games.

Exercise decreased, spending time with friends decreased, travel decreased, and weight increased and became harder to control. Small changes in food intake and a little exercise did not yield the results they used to. Stress increased and came from sources that were very close and important to me. Problems at work, relationship problems, family problems, and sickness and death of people close to me were adding up. Life was becoming more of a chore, not as much a fun adventure or experience. Getting through another day was an accomplishment. Going to bed, I would think that this only meant that tomorrow I had the challenge to survive yet another one. All of my energy seemed to be burned up by simply surviving—continuing to exist. Because of the various stressors I wasn't enjoying those things that I used to.

I had severe financial stress. My family, my job, and my spiritual life no longer brought me the joy and fulfillment that they once had. This was because those were what I had focused my life energy on, and they all ended up being the very things that were causing me the most stress. My blood pressure began to increase. It started to get to levels that were concerning to me. This was very upsetting to me. I have been involved in biofeedback for over twenty years. I felt this should not be happening to me. I should be able to control this.

Both of my parents had a history of hypertension. My father had been in good health most of his life. Later in life he had a couple of mini-strokes, heart disease, and prostate cancer. He died at ninety-eight years of age. He was relatively active until the end.

During the time I was editing this manuscript my mother had a stroke and died at the age of 85. She had still been active, even volunteering at a local daycare center five days per week for four hours per day.

When I started to see my blood pressure increase, it scared me. I started to think, *Am I becoming hypertensive? Am I going to have to take blood pressure medication? Is all that I know about biofeedback and stress management not going to prove to be enough to control my blood pressure?* My weight went up to 205 at one time.

Looking back at that time and how I got through it, I realize that I handled it much better than I might have had I not known what I do about stress and stress management. I wasn't happy during that time, but I was coping. I was able to cope because I was able to regulate how I reacted to the negative things that were happening to and around me. I did my best not to internalize them. I practiced things like muscle relaxation, diaphragmatic breathing, guided imagery, and biofeedback. I was able to reduce the level of negative reactions that my body had to what my mind was dealing with. I don't recall having any symptoms like headaches, neck or back pain, insomnia, or anxiety.

People who knew what I was going through seemed to expect me to be more reactive than I was. Many other people who knew me and spent lots of time around me didn't even know what I was going through or that I was going through anything significant. I believe that I am predisposed to hypertension because of my family history, and the extra weight and lack of enough exercise has also played a part. I am currently working on reducing my blood pressure from many angles, including diet, weight loss, exercise, various modalities of biofeedback, trans cranial electrical stimulation, essential oils like lavender and ocotea, and nutritional supplements. I am studying whatever I can find to increase my knowledge about ways to normalize my blood pressure.

I include this information so that you understand that simply knowing about stress doesn't make you immune to it or the effects of it. You need to do everything you can to combat the negative effects. Also, you should be aware that stress management alone will not necessarily fix all problems that are associated with stress. Stress is often only one of the causes of the symptoms associated with it. Staying with the example of hypertension, you can relax and do biofeedback every day, but if you are genetically prone to hypertension and you eat bacon and eggs for breakfast, a pork sandwich for lunch with a six-pack of beer and potato chips, a big juicy steak with fries and a 20-ounce soda for dinner, and cheesecake for dessert, you will still probably have problems with elevated blood pressure. You still have to work on the other contributing factors even if you manage your stress. That's part of what I had not been doing well. I'm doing much better at it now.

I have been lucky to have learned about biofeedback at such a young age. I was a student at Ossining High School when Adam Crane came to my school to demonstrate biofeedback for my class.

I had always been very interested in science and technology, so when I saw that you could use a piece of equipment to measure how your body was reacting to what you were thinking about, I was immediately hooked. How could this instrument show the fact that a male student was aroused, excited, or embarrassed when asked about his girlfriend?

Adam told our class that he had a job opening and asked for anyone who was interested. I responded right away, along with some others in the class. He picked someone else. I called Adam about that job for weeks and probably months. After telling me over and over that he didn't have a position available anymore, he finally gave in and brought me in for an interview with him; his wife, Dagne; and Marilyn Wexler, who was his receptionist, secretary, office manager, and just about everything else in the business. He hired me, and I started out doing shipping and receiving.

I soon began testing instruments. I have had many other duties since then, including training customers, tech support, sales, internal computer support, and many other things, but I still to this day test instruments. The way that I test them is by connecting them to my body to see if they seem to be working correctly. This means that I am constantly hooked up to biofeedback instruments, so I have the opportunity to do a lot of personal training. I don't think that even I realize the full effect that this has had on me over the years. Think about it; from 1984 through the present I have been hooking myself up to biofeedback instruments of all modalities.

As part of the requirements to become certified as a biofeedback technician by the BCIA (Biofeedback Certification International Alliance), you must experience ten personal training sessions to show that you are able to regulate your own physiology. One of these days I should sit down and attempt to estimate how many personal training sessions I have done on myself. This has helped me to be much more aware of most negative effects stress may be having on my body. I have also learned to recover more quickly from those negative effects. I have often found myself in the middle of stressful situations with other people around me who find it surprising that I am not responding to the situation in the same way that they are. They don't understand how I can be so calm. I have to remind myself that most other people have not had the opportunity to learn about stress management and biofeedback as I have. I'm used to it. It seems like the normal way to react.

When many of the problems that I experienced happened, I wasn't happy about them. I was still upset, but I didn't have as great of a physiological reaction, and it wasn't as long lasting as it might have been without the skills I had learned. I believe that I have the tools to minimize the negative effects that stress can have on my life, and now I want to share the importance of learning them with you.

2 | My Personal Experience with Stress

Chapter 3
_____

Stress and Anger

Anger, or rage, has a large effect on the crime rate. Anger is one of the most important causes of physical crimes against people. This includes crimes like assault, murder, and rape. It is very much underrated as a cause of crime. I say that because more is not being done about it.

Many studies have shown that the majority of criminal offenders come from broken or high-stress families or are the children of violent, angry parents.

The world could be a much nicer place to live if people were able to control anger before or while it is happening.

When some people add to their normal levels of stress and anger abuse of alcohol or lack of sleep, the anger becomes even worse.

Alcohol reduces much needed deep sleep and has a clear effect on people. Some of the aftereffects include irritability and impatience, which often lead to anger. When you don't sleep properly, you tend to have a grumpy, negative attitude. You tend to be less willing to be considerate of others. Alcohol may give temporary relief from problems, but it usually brings more problems. It steals from people the time they need to work on improving themselves. It also can awaken in some people dangerously explosive and even fatal anger and rage. A great number of violent crimes are committed by people who are under the influence of drugs or alcohol.

If you allow yourself to be ruled by anger, you defeat yourself because anger blocks you from reaching your goals.

The level of anger depends on how a person reacts to a stressor. Not everyone will become angry because of the same event. It is how each individual reacts that is important in determining the outcome.

People who are experiencing chronic stress are likely to lose their temper often. The Walker Survey of stress symptoms in farmers shows this. More than 78 percent of the farmers surveyed said that they had become more irritable. Dr. Walter Menninger, a famous psychiatrist, described the highly stressed person as like a volcano about to erupt. Stress can change the easygoing person into one with a short fuse who can suddenly blow up in anger in an even normally mildly upsetting situation. In one example a farmer from Manitoba drove his car through the front door of the local credit union in frustration.

Hardly a week passes that we don't hear a story similar to this.

Chapter 4

Stress in the Workplace

Studies show that people under stress are more likely to have accidents caused by mistakes in judgment, poor perception, and lack of attention.

High levels of chronic stress can cause you to become less efficient and less able to adjust to changing situations. They can also cause you to miss out on many of the little pleasures that other people enjoy every day.

Research by Töres Theorell and Robert Karasek has shown a clear relationship between increased job stress and cardiovascular disease. For more on the subject, you can read *Healthy Work: Stress, Productivity, and the Reconstruction of Working Life* by Robert Karasek and Töres Theorell.

Stress can be a big problem in the workplace in many ways. It can cause problems for the workers as well as the company owners.

Let's look at an example of a business that sells products or services. Many things can affect the sales totals of a company—the product, the marketing and advertising, and the performance of the salespeople themselves. I want to consider just the performance of the sales force. The sales force is made up of people, not machines.

Many things, including stress, can affect humans. Each person on the sales force has a certain performance and production potential. Every one of them has the capability to perform at 100 percent.

Let us say that when one of the salespeople performs at 100 percent, he or she produces $50,000 per month gross, and his/her commission of 10 percent is $5,000. Now let us say that under moderate stress he or she only performs at 75 percent due to lack of focus, time spent thinking about problems, and inefficient breathing, which causes less oxygen to the brain, affecting thinking. Increased muscle tension causes pain in the neck, shoulders, and back, as well as headaches.

Now the salesperson is paying attention to pain some of the time instead of work. He or she may also have stomach and digestive problems. This can lead to more time in the bathroom and more time lost because of attention to stomach pain. The salesperson with these problems may start to take longer coffee breaks and longer lunch breaks. He or she may make more personal phone calls. He or she may feel less motivated to make the next sales call. He or she tends to be less effective on the calls that are made. He or she may end up missing more days at work due to real or faked sickness.

In this example, if the salesperson is only performing at 75 percent, the sales gross falls from $50,000 to $37,000. The commission falls from $5,000 to $3,700. The loss to the company gross is $12,500. The personal loss to the salesperson in commission is $1,250.

Businesspeople understand dollars and cents. Multiply this by the number of people in a company's entire sales force. Is it important for a business to help its employees deal with stress? What if the performance dropped to even lower than 75 percent? The losses would be even greater. We all have had times that we were at work while we were dealing with some kind of stress. At times we tend to just go through the motions, knowing that we are not performing at 100 percent. The quality of our work suffers. Sometimes we might not even go to work if we believe that the effects of the stress are too much for us to deal with.

Absenteeism due to job stress has escalated.

According to a survey of 800,000 workers in more than 300 companies, the number of workers calling in sick due to stress increased by 300 percent from 1996 to 2000. It has been estimated that 1 million workers miss work every day because of stress. The European Agency for Safety and Health at Work reported that more than half of the 550 million working days lost every year in the United States due to absenteeism are related to stress and that 20 percent of all last-minute no-shows are due to job stress. If this happens with key employees, it can have an effect that spreads down the line to disrupt the whole operation. Unforeseen absenteeism is estimated to cost US companies $602 per worker per year, and the cost for large companies could be as high as $3.5 million per year. A 1997 three-year study done by one large company found that 60 percent of employee absences could be traced to psychological problems because of job stress.

Work Stress Statistics

- 40 percent of job turnover is due to stress.

- Replacing an average employee today costs between $3,000 and $13,000.

- 60 to 80 percent of accidents on the job are stress related, and some, like the Three Mile Island and Exxon Valdez disasters, can affect many thousands very far away.

- In California the number of workers' compensation claims for mental stress increased by almost 700 percent over eight years, and 90 percent were successful, with an average award of $15,000.

- Increases in workers' compensation premiums every year as a result of mental stress claims threaten to bankrupt the system in several states.

- Studies show that keyboard entry operators who are under stress (because they are not sure if their activities are being monitored for performance evaluation) have a much higher incidence of these complaints and injuries.

In the 2000 annual Attitudes in the American Workplace VI poll, sponsored by the Marlin Company, it was reported that:

- 80 percent of workers experience stress on the job, almost half say they could use help in learning how to deal with stress, and 42 percent believe that their coworkers need help too;

- 14 percent of those who responded had felt like hitting a coworker in the past year but didn't;

- 25 percent had felt like screaming or yelling because of job stress;

- 10 percent are worried about a person at work they believe could become violent

- 9 percent know of an assault or violent act that happened in their workplace; and

- 18 percent had experienced some kind of threat or verbal intimidation in the past year.

The 2000 Integra Survey reported that:

- 65 percent of workers said that workplace stress had caused problems, and more than 10 percent said that the problems had major effects;

- 10 percent said they worked in an atmosphere where physical violence had occurred because of job stress, and in this group, 42 percent reported that yelling and other verbal abuse was common;

- 29 percent had yelled at coworkers because of workplace stress, 14 percent said that equipment has been damaged because of workplace rage, and 2 percent admitted that they had actually personally hit someone;

- 19 percent or almost one out of five respondents had quit a previous position because of job stress, and nearly one quarter have been driven to tears because of workplace stress;

- 62 percent often ended the day with work-related neck pain, 44 percent reported stressed-out eyes, 38 percent complained of painful hands, and 34 percent reported trouble sleeping because they were too stressed out;

- 12 percent had called in sick because of job stress; and

- more than 50 percent said they often spent twelve-hour days on work-related duties, and an equal number frequently skipped lunch because of the stress of job demands.

Workplace Accidents

Mistakes cost money, injury, and loss of life.

The greatest cause of lost productive years of life is accidents. Almost one million productive-person hours are lost every year due to work-related accidents. Work accidents are very expensive to the employer. Yearly accident costs are estimated to be $31.4 billion in lost wages, medical and insurance expenses, and property damage in the United States alone (National Safety Council 1983).

There has been a lot of research on work accidents, including behavioral and physiological models. The causes and the reasons of accidents can be separated into two categories, direct and indirect in general. Indirect causes can be classified into two major categories: environmental factors (unsafe chemical, physical, or mechanical conditions) and personal factors. Major environmental or technical causes can be due to failure by management to put in place and oversee safety procedures, unsatisfactory maintenance of plant, insufficient or ineffective safety devices on machinery, unusual wear and tear, lack of preventive maintenance, and so on.

Automation is not a solution for work accidents that are caused by technical reasons. This is the reason why human error is an important factor.

The majority of work accidents are due to a combination of unsafe physical conditions and unsafe acts, and most accidents arise from human error. Some studies showed that 85 to 90 percent of all injuries were caused by human error and only 10 to 15 percent by hazardous conditions. In other words for every four accidents caused by human deficiencies, one is caused by technical or mechanical defects. For example, about 70 percent of aircraft accidents and incidents have been caused by human error, and the importance of human error as a major factor is now universally recognized. It is of course impossible to create a completely safe work environment where no one could possibly hurt themselves.

Most accidents happen because of a problem with the operator or personal behavior rather than the machine itself. To reduce work accidents, it is important to identify the cause of the human errors.

Anything that might cause a person to operate equipment unsafely should be examined. This includes accident proneness, aggression, difficulty adjusting socially, impulsivity, risk taking, age and experience, insufficient education, duration of work, and stress.

No two people react in the same way to a stressful event; one may become withdrawn and depressed, while another may be hyperactive, compulsive, or abnormally outgoing; one sleeps too much, and another develops insomnia (Stranks and Dewis 1986). Any of these behavioral reactions to stress can cause a work-related accident.

This is a very good reason that businesses should look at incorporating stress management programs. They should automatically be part of any Employment Assistance Program (EAP).

Some of the psychological effects of stress are hardly noticeable. This may be true in cases of chronic fatigue. Over time the mind/ body can be overwhelmed and drained by chronic stress. This state of exhaustion eventually has a negative effect on our moods. When people feel tired and run-down, they become somewhat depressed, lose interest in things that they used to enjoy, don't spend time with their friends, and get much less happiness and satisfaction out of life. Your attention span may be decreased, and your desire and energy to get things done and explore new ideas may be lower. It is very important to notice these signals even though they may not seem important. These very symptoms are signs that stress is doing damage. The sooner you notice and do something about it, the less damage will be done.

When you react to stress in a negative way, it can have effects on your ability to think clearly and focus. High beta brainwaves, which are associated with overthinking, obsessing, and anxiety, increase in power when the brain is reacting to stress. This makes it difficult for a person to think clearly. Though the slightly slower beta brainwaves are appropriate for active thinking, the high beta waves are not healthy in high amplitude for any long period of time. The brain can run more efficiently if the power is higher at a lower frequency like low beta or even alpha when a person is not involved in an active thinking activity. The brain causes chemicals to be produced that help to heal and repair the body, while there is more power in the slower brainwaves like alpha and theta while awake, and theta and delta while a person is sleeping. The brain causes chemicals to be produced that can cause damage to the body when there is too much fast brainwave activity (high beta) for long periods of time. See the list for the various brainwaves and associated mind states.

Types of Brainwaves

- Delta 1–4 Hz: deep sleep

- Theta 4–7 Hz: creativity, inattention, daydreaming, depression

- Alpha 8–12 Hz: meditation, inner calm, peacefulness

- SMR 12–15 Hz: state of being internally oriented, stillness, relaxed thought

- Beta 13–21 Hz: focused, active thinking

- High Beta 20–32 Hz: anxiety, overthinking, OCD

Bruce McEwen, PhD, is head of the neuroendocrinology laboratory at Rockefeller University in New York. He has done research that shows that long-term stress is an important factor in the development of progressive memory loss.

Dr. McEwen suggests that repeated stress can cause the body to develop an inability to turn off its major biological stress pathway. This can directly lead to substantial memory loss. This information was reported in a January 15, 1998, *New England Journal of Medicine* article.

Two mechanisms were suggested. First, stress increases the secretion of cortisol by the adrenal gland that directly slows down short-term memory function in the hippocampus area of the brain. If the brain continues to sense stress, glucocorticoids (the body's natural steroids) and excitatory amino acid neurotransmitters (the chemicals that cause nerve transmissions) are produces and directly result in atrophy or wasting away of nerve fibers in the hippocampus.

If the stress is short-term, then the memory loss is reversible. If, on the other hand, it is long-term (months to years), the damaged brain neurons die and do not grow back.

This constant wear and tear on the brain due to chronic stress is frightening. That is the negative. On the positive side, it is possible to actively prevent nerve cell loss in our brains. If you have been forgetful lately, and you are under a great deal of stress, you should start working on stress management to reduce and perhaps reverse the damage.

Chapter 5

Attention

I believe that ADD/ADHD is becoming an easy way to label and deal with many people, especially children, who don't neatly fit into the way that we do things in our society. I am sure that there are many cases that really should be diagnosed as a medical disorder. I also believe that much of what is being called ADD/ADHD is a result of the environment that we now live in.

According to an article in *The Chronicle of Higher Education* titled "The Net Generation Goes to College," by Scott Carlson, "Tech-savvy 'Millennials' have lots of gadgets, like to multitask, and expect to control what, when, and how they learn. Should colleges cater to them?" "Change your teaching style. Make blogs, iPods, and video games part of your pedagogy. And learn to accept divided attention spans. A new generation of students has arrived—and sorry, but they might not want to hear you lecture for an hour." That is the message of Richard T. Sweeney, University Librarian of the Robert W. Van Houten Library of New Jersey Institute of Technology.

Issues of attention and multitasking are also discussed in a paper titled "Confronting the Challenges of Participatory Culture: Media Education for the 21st Century," by Henry Jenkins, Director of the Comparative Media Studies Program at the Massachusetts Institute of Technology.

Watching TV is not what it used to be. Have you noticed how short the segments are during commercials, TV shows, or movies? The camera is constantly switching views, usually every few seconds. Music videos are the same. This is training our minds/brains to expect to switch from one subject to another very quickly. School learning is not like that. Business learning is usually not like that. Most learning is not like that. Most learning involves staying with one subject for a relatively long period of time. No wonder many children who spend lots of time watching TV or playing fast-moving, complex video games become bored when they are expected to sit in a classroom and listen to a teacher talk about one thing for thirty minutes or more straight.

Listening to the radio has become a chore to me too. Most radio stations play the same songs over and over. I think that this has a conditioning effect. People who really don't seem to be very talented are made into megastars. People hear their songs on the radio over and over. They see their music videos on TV. They end up going to the store and buying their CD or downloading it from iTunes or a similar online service.

There is no downtime when you aren't doing anything. There is no quiet time. Enjoying nature is not encouraged. People are always going, doing something. The title of a book comes to mind— *Don't Just Do Something, Sit There: A Mindfulness Retreat*, by Sylvia Boorstein. This book describes taking a real break from the fast pace of life to quiet your mind. It also talks about the tremendous values that can be gained from doing so.

Remember Pong? It just had one knob that you turned clockwise or counterclockwise to control the paddle. That was all. New video games have lots of buttons on the controller and action on the screen. Keeping the brain/mind occupied, processing information. This doesn't give us a chance to even know what we think about anything. We are constantly fed what to think by others. No time to plan. No time to meditate.

TV watching is up. According to a 2012 Nielsen survey, the average person in the United States of America watches more than thirty-four hours of TV every week. This adds up to over two months of nonstop TV-watching per year. Over a sixty-five-year lifetime, that totals over nine years of watching TV. There are so many TV channels to choose from. There is always something to watch on TV. You can also add to this, programs that we DVR and watch later, YouTube, and other content we watch on the Internet on our PC, phone, or tablet. We are suffering from information overload. There is more than enough information but not enough time or skill to process it and choose/select which information is valuable.

Learning to manage stress and information overload can help to improve attention and focus. The brain is capable of processing amazing amounts of data, but it also needs to rest so that it can perform more efficiently.

Chapter 6

Sports and Performance

Just as stress can affect work performance on the job, as discussed earlier, stress can also affect performance in sports, music, and the military.

Most of these types of activities are only different from everyday jobs in that they usually require performing at extraordinary levels. People who are not better than average in sports, music, and acting don't tend to make a living at it. People who don't perform better than average in the military don't tend to rise to higher levels.

Athletes must be talented; they must exercise, study, and practice in order to be chosen to play and to do well. Sports are full of stressful situations. There is the pressure of winning, other athletes ready and waiting to take your place, concern about injury, pressure from coaches, pressure from fans, pressure from the media, pressure from friends and family, and of course pressure from athletes themselves. If an athlete is not doing well, then there is pressure to do better or possibly lose his or her playing time or position altogether. If the athlete is doing well, then there is pressure to continue doing well or to do even better. There are moments of pressure before and during performance and then again after performance, with interviews and preparation for the next time.

An athlete cannot just learn to stay totally relaxed throughout his or her performance. He or she wouldn't be any good. It wouldn't work. Most sports require vigorous physical activity at times, including lots of muscle contraction. You cannot keep all of your muscles relaxed while you swing a baseball bat or tennis racquet, throw a football, kick a soccer ball, or punch another boxer. You cannot be in a deep meditative state during the active periods of these sports either. Most physical sports require intense physical and mental activity. There are times, however, when athletes can relax their minds and bodies. Athletes can relax before the time for them to perform. This can help them to prepare. They can relax and go through in their minds successfully performing when the time comes to do so. They can often relax during timeouts and rest periods. Even if they have to stay focused mentally, they can relax somewhat physically so that they are not wearing themselves out while they are supposed to be resting. Athletes can keep their muscles relaxed until it is time to perform, and then they may tense their muscles much more than a nonathlete would be able to if he or she tried. The key is learning to be "in the moment."

The person who is able to keep his or her cool during sports is often able to win. Many players "talk trash" to their opponents to get them upset because they know that most players don't perform as well when they are upset. Muhammad Ali, Kevin Garnet, Larry Bird, and Deion Sanders are a few examples of top trash talkers in sports.

Many times an athlete has problems in mind that have nothing to do with the sport, which causes stress, distraction, and less mental focus. This can of course affect performance negatively. A great example of this is Tiger Woods. Before the news of his personal problems became public, he was on top of the golf world. Since the news came out, he has been doing terrible compared to before. He went through public embarrassment and criticism, a very expensive divorce settlement, and the loss of full custody of his children. How is that for stress and what it can do to your performance in sports?

Many times a talented athlete "chokes" even though he or she is naturally talented and well prepared. This can also be due to stress and loss of focus.

Many more athletes are starting to use sports psychologists and biofeedback to help them deal with stress and learn self-control over their minds and bodies.

Timothy Harkness, a counseling psychologist, trained shooter Abhinav Bindra with about 150 hours of biofeedback as part of his preparation for the Beijing Olympics, where he won a gold medal in the 10-meter men's air rifle event.

The Italian soccer team AC-Milan trained using biofeedback by Bruno De Michelis, the head of sport science, and won the 2006 World Cup soccer tournament. They set up what they called the Mind Room, where they had several Thought Technology biofeedback systems set up. The athletes used this equipment to practice relaxation and self-regulation on surface EMG, skin temperature, skin conductance, respiration, heart rate, and EEG (brainwave) biofeedback.

Dr. Vietta "Sue" Wilson is a well-known sports psychologist who has worked with many pro, Olympic, and student athletes. She was recognized at the 2005 Association for the Advancement of Applied Sport conference for her work.

Erik Peper, PhD, is another well-known psychologist who uses biofeedback to help athletes with performance issues.

Stress and tension can also be a problem for musicians. Many musicians practice very hard and have lots of pressure on them to do well. As they perform some of them hold excess muscle tension in their hands, fingers, shoulders, neck, mouth, and other areas. This works against them as they perform. Playing an instrument requires fine muscle control. When you hold excess tension in your muscles, fine control becomes more difficult. Some therapists have also developed special biofeedback equipment and protocols to help musicians with this type of problem.

In the military, as you can imagine, there is a lot of stress. There is a great deal of stress from the very beginning for people who serve in the military. From the time a new recruit signs the papers there is stress. There is the thought of being separated from family and friends. There is basic training. Some are deployed, and some experience combat. This covers the full range of anticipatory stress to full-blown severe stress and PTSD, post-traumatic stress disorder.

Those service people who experience combat also may have to deal with losing some of those who fought with them. After military service people finally return home, their stress is usually not over. There are often problems at work and home when they return.

They may have trouble dealing with the things that they have experienced. They may not be able to share their experiences with the people that they come home to. They may have trouble sleeping and nightmares. They may be overly vigilant. Relationships can be strained due to symptoms and personality changes.

Imagine a situation where a soldier has returned home from combat safely. His family welcomes him home after he has been away for many months. While he was deployed, he was involved in combat. Several of his friends were injured and some killed. He also may have killed enemy combatants as well as possibly some innocent civilians. Finally he is sent home. He has feelings of guilt because others were injured or killed but he gets to go home safe. He has feelings of guilt for some of what he has done. He is haunted by some of the things that he has seen. Now, when he comes home, his family and friends expect him to pick up where he left off. They expect him to be the same person he was before he left. He is not the same person. He has a lot of stress to deal with. His friends and family may not understand the extent of what he is dealing with because he doesn't feel that he can tell them.

Chapter 7

Stress and Crime

According to two studies, the United States has the unfortunate distinction of having the highest violent crime rate of any industrialized country. On average about twenty people are killed at work every week in the United States, making murder the second-highest cause of workplace deaths overall and the leading one for women. Each week 18,000 nonfatal violent crimes, such as sexual and other assaults, also take place while the victims are at work. That is about one million per year. The numbers are probably even higher because many incidents are not even reported.

Some dangerous occupations like police officers and cab drivers normally have higher rates of homicide and nonfatal assaults. This is understandable. Not so understandably, postal workers who work in a relatively safe environment have experienced so many deaths due to job stress that "going postal" has become part of our language. "Desk rage" and "phone rage" have also become common terms. There are now many video clips showing people "losing it" at work. Just do a search on YouTube.

As social media has become a part of how people interact, it has also become a place where people are bullied and humiliated. There have even been a number of suicides attributed to information posted on social media. We have also had a growing number of shootings at schools.

How many times have you heard something like this? A report on the news talking about a horrible murder, conducting an interview, asks a neighbor about the perpetrator/suspect. The neighbor says, "He was a very nice person, quiet. He never bothered anybody…" Very often this is how people describe a murder suspect. Many times he or she is probably just a normal person, with the same negative tendencies and character flaws that we all have, pushed past his or her personal limit of stress. He or she loses it and acts irrationally.

Remember the 1993 movie *Falling Down* starring Michael Douglas? I challenge you to think honestly. How many times have we all felt like we could kill somebody or at least cause somebody serious physical harm? We just don't do it. We maintain control. We don't reach our boiling points. This is probably due to whatever stress management skills we already have. How much better could our lives be if we increased our skill at managing stress?

At the time I wrote this section of the book, there was a relevant story in the news. We had recently experienced one of the most devastating natural disasters in the history of the United States of America: Hurricane Katrina. New Orleans was one of the hardest hit areas. Besides the deaths and physical damage to homes, businesses, and infrastructure, this storm caused a devastating amount of stress to the nation, but more specifically the people who were directly affected. People lost their homes, businesses, jobs, cars, other possessions, loved ones, and hope for the future. At the convention center and Superdome stadium, some people watched people die right before their eyes waiting for help. There were also reports of people who were attacked and/or raped while waiting for help to arrive. There were reports of people seeing babies born without medical assistance. It was reported that some of the babies died because they didn't have the medical care they needed. Older people and sick people at hospitals and nursing homes were left to die because help didn't arrive in time for them. People saw things that they would normally have never seen. They were not prepared to experience these types of things. Some of those affected by the stress were the police. They also were not prepared to experience these things at such a magnitude. They also lived in the area and lost the same things that others lost. One report claimed that 75 percent of the police force had lost their homes. Many of them did not report for work or walked off the job. The police chief resigned, probably because of stress about the enormous pressure that was placed on him.

During this time a group of about four policemen were caught on video savagely beating an older African-American man who was a retired school teacher. He was over sixty years old. They claimed that he was drunk and disorderly in public. The man claimed that he was not drunk and that he has not been drinking alcohol for many years. He apparently got into an argument with one of the officers that just got out of control. The video showed two officers holding the man with his face against a wall while another officer punched the man repeatedly in the back of the head. They then brought him down to the ground. One of the officers was holding him by the foot and twisting his foot and leg as he lay facedown on the pavement. A later video showed him lying there face down in a pool of blood. I didn't see anything in the video that showed that the man offered anything that could be considered serious resistance that would have required anywhere near such force.

Another officer was seen in the video confronting one of the media people who were involved in videotaping the incident. He grabbed the man, who was backing up and showing his media credential badge to the officer. He pushed him up against a vehicle as he yelled at him. He was saying something to the effect of "You don't know what we are dealing with here. I have been down here every day dealing with this and you just come down here and think you know everything. Why don't you go home?"

The officers were arrested, and I believe that they were charged with assault. The officers plead not guilty! I believe that an assault charge is much less than what is called for, but this is not the purpose of me bringing up the story. As the media reported on the story, I heard a few times that questions were being asked as to whether stress played a role in why the officers beat the man as they did. I do believe that stress played a huge role. I don't think that it is a valid excuse at all though. I believe that they were acting out something that was in their hearts. I believe that they may have been able to suppress the urge to act out such an attack had they not been under the extreme stress that they were dealing with. Even though stress may have pushed them to the point of acting in that way, they should still be held accountable for their actions.

I believe that if law enforcement officers received stress management training there would be fewer excessive force problems. I don't think they would be nonexistent, but I believe that they would drop significantly. Some officers might be afraid that stress management training would make them too mellow to do their job effectively. I don't believe that the stress management training would have any negative effects on the performance of the officers. I believe that their performance would actually improve. It would make them more aware, more focused, and more able to adapt to quick-changing circumstances. I believe that they would be less likely to freeze during emergency situations. They would be more able to assess the situation quickly and act accordingly. They would be less likely to underreact and less likely to overreact. Burnout can be a big problem with all types of law enforcement. Stress management should automatically be an ongoing part of the training for officers.

I believe that stress often plays a part in many crime situations. People lose their ability to stop aberrant thoughts and urges from turning into actions when they are under stress and don't have or don't use the stress management skills that could help them avoid crossing the line. Many people have thought about stealing money, beating somebody up, or even killing a person who has done them wrong. Most of the time people decide not to do those things. They are able to stop themselves from actually doing what comes to their thoughts. When this type of inhibition doesn't work, a person may "snap" and do what is out of character for them.

Many crimes happen at home because of stress. Child abuse and spousal abuse are often triggered by unmanaged stress. A parent may be upset because of problems that have nothing to do with his or her child. He or she may have financial, job, relationship, or other problems causing stress. He or she may become aggressive and violent toward the child to release some of the negative energy. The same thing can happen with a husband becoming aggressive and violent with his wife. (In some cases it is the wife becoming aggressive and violent with her husband).

Why do thieves steal? For some it is that they have financial need. Their financial problems may have become so serious that they are now a great source of stress. When this happens, a person may not think clearly enough to see other alternatives without the potential problems that go along with stealing. Stealing is an option, but it has some very negative consequences, especially if the person gets caught. If caught a person can suffer humiliation, go to prison, and lose his or her job, home, and family. When a person is calm enough under the same financial stress, he or she may consider the risks and decide to look for other options. If he or she is affected by stress, he or she may not think clearly enough to consider the risks. He or she may be suffering from tunnel vision, seeing stealing as the only option. The same could be said about selling drugs.

According to an article from the Natural Law Party (www.natural-law.org/platform/crime.html), crime costs Americans $450 billion every year. Tougher laws and sentences have not really helped. Violent youth crimes and gang activity are growing problems. Young people in the United States are twelve times more likely to be killed by guns than in other countries.

According to the National Center for Juvenile Justice (1995), the murder rate among fourteen- to seventeen-year-olds increased 165 percent during the last 10 years, and the number of arrests for violent crime among ten- to seventeen-year-olds doubled. In addition, according to *USA Today* (November 13, 1995), the number of teenage arrests on weapons charges has doubled since 1985.

The article states that tough policy is not enough. Effective crime prevention measures are crucial. Putting people who commit crimes in prison isolates them from society, but it doesn't get rid of the reasons for the crime.

Here is a direct quote from the article: "Most violent crime is 'an impulsive response to an immediate stressful situation,' often committed under the influence of drugs or alcohol—not a rational, considered action."

The Natural Law Party believes that standard methods of dealing with crime don't work because they don't hit the root of the problem, which they are convinced is the "epidemic" of stress in our society.

Medical science has documented that over the past twenty years, this stress in our society has caused stress-related sicknesses, including high blood pressure, stroke, and heart disease. This stress also causes sickness in society, including drug abuse, violence, and crime.

Crime prevention programs should include a focus on the psychological and physiological problems caused by long-term traumatic stress. Stress can cause the nervous system to become out of balance due to psychophysiological reactions. One of the stress chemicals that can be overproduced is cortisol. Lower than normal levels of serotonin are produced during a stress reaction. When the body is out of balance like this, a person can become anxious, fearful, angry, and susceptible to impulsive violent behavior and drug abuse.

When many or most of the people who make up society are stressed, a general stressful atmosphere is created throughout the community. This tense atmosphere sets the table for crime and violence. Reducing stress in individuals (especially those at high risk) and throughout society can serve to reduce crime.

More than forty studies have been published that have shown that when large numbers of people practiced Transcendental Meditation in a specific area there was a reduction in social stress and violence.

The studies have shown there to be an effect on the surrounding communities. There were reductions in crime and deaths from war. There were also improvements in the economies and the mood of those in the community.

Rehabilitation of people in prison is very important for preventing crime since about 90 percent of those in prison will be released at some time. They are at a higher risk of committing crime than people who were never in prison before.

The evidence from a five-year study showed that a Transcendental Meditation program put in place in a high-security prison decreased violence and return of inmates to prison. The inmates learned to relax. This had the effect of decreasing their stress and aggressiveness. It also helped with mental problems.

The environment that people live in can itself be stressful and contribute to crime. Many city areas are overcrowded. The apartment buildings (sometimes referred to as the projects) are run-down, dirty, and in need of repairs and upgrades. The surrounding houses and businesses are usually also run-down. There are also usually abandoned houses and buildings in the area. The parks and other community activity centers are often in buildings that are in very bad shape, so people don't even bother trying to use them. With few positive activities to become involved in and a lack of jobs, both youth and adults are at higher risk of turning to crime.

Another article titled "The Root Causes of Crime" (CS&CPC Statement on the Root Causes of Crime, approved in 1996) says, "Crime is primarily the outcome of multiple adverse social, economic, cultural and family conditions."

It lists these categories:

Economic Factors/Poverty

Social Environment

Family Structures

Under Family Structures it says "Dysfunctional family conditions contribute to future delinquency."

Family structure problems listed are:

Parental inadequacy

Parental conflict

Parental criminality

Lack of communication (both in quality and quantity)

Lack of respect and responsibility

Abuse and neglect of children

Family violence

These are all obvious sources of *stress*.

The article states that stress during pregnancy can even have negative effects on fetal development, which can lead to slow development, neurological problems, and later behavior problems in children.

Those people who do commit crimes have increased difficulty in getting employment, which increases the chances that they will turn to crime once again to get money.

Another crime fact listed in the article is that over half of young violent criminals had seen the wife physically abused in the home they lived in.

Stress and Disasters

Both man-made and natural disasters are huge sources of stress. One of our most recent local examples of this was Super Storm Sandy. A *New York Daily News* article from May 23, 2013 reported that post-traumatic stress disorder had become a big problem in the aftermath of the storm. People have reported symptoms including suicidal thoughts, strained marriages, emotional stress, depression, sadness, anxiety, anger, and drug and alcohol abuse. Other examples of stressful disasters include the many school shootings, wars, tsunamis, earthquakes, floods, wildfires, tornadoes, explosions, the 911 attacks, and nuclear accidents. Therapists and trauma experts attempt to help many of the survivors at least initially, but what is the ongoing effect on the survivors? Do the people that they interact with even know what they have been through? Do they take that into consideration when dealing with them? How do they go on having experienced what they experienced? What are they doing to manage the stress? What is the long-term effect if the stress is not managed?

Chapter 8

Nutrition and Stress

It is important to know that what you eat can affect your stress level.

Not eating enough or not eating enough healthy foods can cause imbalances in your blood sugar level. These fluctuations can lead to mood swings, fatigue, and poor concentration.

Too much caffeine can lead to poor concentration and decreased effectiveness, sleep disturbances, and increased levels of cortisol in the blood, as well as other negative effects.

Poor nutrition can also lead to lowered immunity so you're more susceptible to illnesses, both minor and major. As you can imagine, this can lead to other problems, including increased stress levels.

Foods That Cause Stress

Caffeine

Found in coffee, tea, colas, and chocolates. Caffeine increases stress levels because it stimulates the central nervous system. Too much caffeine intake can cause a hyperactive mood, irritation, and stress.

Alcohol

Alcohol, in large amounts, can disrupt sleep. Heavy use of alcohol can create interpersonal problems with family, friends, and coworkers. This can generate many sources of stress.

Sugar

Sugar increases the energy levels in the body short-term. Unfortunately, the final effect is negative. The reason is that the body deals with sugar by releasing insulin into the bloodstream to reduce the sugar level. The increase in insulin often continues even after the body has processed the sugar. This can cause a drop in energy level.

Foods That Reduce Stress

Proteins

Proteins maintain the body's muscles, strengthen them, and help in fighting stress. Some examples of foods that are rich in protein are meat, chicken, fish, eggs, cheese, milk, beans, and soy.

Carbohydrates

Carbohydrates that are eaten in an unrefined form will boost positive energy levels and therefore help reduce stress. Some examples are whole grain bread and pasta, brown rice, vegetables, fruits, etc.

Potassium

Potassium helps prevent high blood pressure. Corn, potatoes, avocados, leeks, fish, natural yogurt, chicken, and bananas contain lots of potassium.

Iron

Iron helps in moving oxygen through the bloodstream. Lack of enough iron can lead to poor brain function. This in turn weakens the body's stress-response levels. Some foods that are rich in iron are eggs, lean meat, dried fruits, whole grain cereals, peas, and potatoes.

Zinc and Copper

Zinc helps to speed the breakdown process of proteins. This slows proteins from being converted to fat. Some studies show that a lack of copper in the body can harm the heart. Foods like chicken, liver, kidney, oysters, banana, rice, beans, pears, and soy contain zinc and copper.

Chapter 9

Stress at Home

Have you ever been told that you have a short fuse? What does having a short fuse really mean? It means that you have allowed your stress level to build up to the point that even a small additional stress causes you to "lose it"—lose control and react irrationally. Sometimes when you are already under stress you may overreact to something small. This can confuse and surprise people who are around you because your reaction is so unreasonable and out of balance to the event.

Here is one example. A father comes home from a very stressful day at work. He is not making enough money to keep up with his bills. He is in debt and doesn't know how he is going to make the mortgage payment this month. As soon as he walks through the door, one of his children asks him for a dollar. His reaction is to slap the child across the room, yell that he or she is always asking him for money, and storm out of the room. This type of poor reaction to stress can and usually does lead to even more stress. Now he may have a fight with his wife about hitting the child. He might even get arrested, lose time at work, and even lose his job because of the arrest. Now he has made his situation much worse. He has also strained his relationship with his child. It will cost him way more than the dollar that the child asked him for. Learning even the most basic stress management skills and using them could help you avoid these types of problems. Practicing stress management techniques before, during, and/or after stressful events can bring your stress level back down to a manageable level so the next stressful event won't bring you to your boiling point. You will tend to react more normally and be less likely to overreact or "lose it."

Chapter 10

Community

Stewart Wolf presented a lecture titled "The Scales of Libra: Social Factors That Influence Stress" at The First International Congress on Stress. In it he discussed a twenty-five-year follow-up to a study of a small town in Pennsylvania called Roseto. The study showed that there are very strong cardiovascular health benefits of living in a community with close social support. He predicted that as time went on and those who lived in Roseto began to give up their social lifestyle traditions, those health benefits would diminish. At the beginning of his research, Roseto had one of the lowest cardiovascular-related death rates in the United States. It was not attributed to lower cholesterol, blood pressure, or habits like smoking, eating, or exercise. What was different, according to Wolf, was the kind of community it was. They were mostly Italian descendants whose ancestors had come from the same small area in Italy about a hundred years before. They had chosen the site to settle because it was very similar to where they had come from in Italy. The people of Roseto continued the same values and basic way of life of their ancestors. The older people of the community were looked up to, cared for, and respected. They were seen as a resource for things like advice. It was common for children, parents, and grandparents to live in the same house. It was rare for any of the elderly to be placed in a nursing home. They were not materialistic. Any shows of wealth or status like houses, cars, clothes, etc., were frowned on. Most of the people married within their own faith. They followed the tradition of naming their first child after a grandparent. The people of Roseto were friendly and kind. Families and friends got together often to celebrate things like birthdays, anniversaries, or children's first communions.

In 1963 Wolf predicted that the people of Roseto would move away from their old ways and begin to lose the related cardiovascular health benefits. He started to see the changes and associated effects by 1970. People started to build fancy houses and buy expensive cars. They started to marry outside of their religion and community. The tradition of naming after a grandparent lost popularity. Participation in local social events like men's clubs and church decreased. The elderly lost the prominent place they once held.

Along with the societal changes, Wolf also saw an increase in heart attack deaths in Roseto as heart attack deaths in the rest of the country were decreasing. There was more than a 100 percent increase in coronary heart disease, a 300 percent increase in hypertension, and a large increase in strokes, even though the citizens were smoking less and eating less fat. His prediction was correct. He was not surprised. He noted that a Dr. C.P. Donosson had written about a similar effect fifty years before in his book *Civilization and Disease.* Donosson had seen that in remote areas of Africa with a more ancient society there were no hypertension, diabetes, or peptic ulcer problems. These and other stress-related illnesses grew quickly after the "Western" ways were brought in.

In the book *Cancer Stress and Death,* the Nobel Prize winner it was reported that Albert Schweitzer noted that when he went to Gabon, a west central African country, in 1913, he didn't see any cancer cases. As years passed he saw the beginning of cancer cases, and the numbers increased. He was led to believe that this was due to the natives of Gabon being influenced to live more like the whites who came in.

Another example is from the observations of anthropologist and Arctic explorer Vilhjalmur Stefansson, who in his book *Cancer: Disease of Civilization?* stated that he didn't see any cancer in the Eskimos he saw when he first got to the Arctic, but he started to see an increase in cases in the Eskimos over time as they gained closer contact with white civilization. Sir Robert McCarrison was a doctor who studied Hunza natives in Kashmir from 1904 to 1911. He saw no cases of cancer there. The Hunza natives also lived extraordinarily long. McCarrison concluded that this was because they were "far removed from the refinement of civilization and endowed with a nervous system of notable stability."

These stories suggest that a sense of belonging and strong social support can provide protection from the negative health effects of stress. It also shows that societal stress, not only cholesterol and fat intake, plays a role in the onset of coronary heart disease.

As more people become aware of the negative effects of stress, we can begin to make a difference in the health and quality of life in our communities. The greater the number of people practicing stress management, the greater will be the positive effects on communities around the world.

Chapter 11

Physical Symptoms

"What happens in the mind of man is always reflected in the disease of his body." – René Dubos

Many symptoms can be caused by stress, including tension headaches, neck pain, back pain, and ulcers. Some existing conditions can be made worse by stress, including asthma, hypertension, diabetes, and pain.

Back on June 6, 1983, *Time* ran a cover story titled "Stress, the Epidemic of the Eighties." The author said that it was our biggest health problem. I don't think it has improved at all. There is reason to believe that it is much worse now. Surveys show that people in the United States believe that they are more stressed now than they were ten or twenty years ago.

There is evidence that the "type A" behavior is as powerful a risk factor for coronary heart disease as high cholesterol, hypertension, and cigarette smoking, according to the work of Meyer Friedman and Ray Rosenman. See *Type A Behavior and Your Heart*, 1974, Meyer Friedman and Ray Rosenman.

According to Daniel Goleman, PhD, author of the books *Emotional Intelligence* and *Destructive Emotions* and *New York Times* contributor on behavioral and brain sciences, people with chronic anxiety and high stress have double the risk of disease.

In a 2004 interview on Shareguide.com, a holistic health magazine and resource directory, Dr. Goleman suggested that stress is about as much a factor in heart attack, stroke, and other serious illnesses as high cholesterol or high blood pressure. He also suggested that stress can have about the same impact as smoking or poor diet. It is not good enough to not smoke, exercise, and eat the proper foods. We still need to address the problem of unmanaged stress. Dr. Goldman also describes anger as the emotion that is most harmful to the heart. He believes that anger management and therapy should be part of treatment for patients with heart disease.

He stated that people who tend to be often angry and or aggravated in their early lives are much more likely to die in their forties and fifties from heart disease, as well as all other causes.

Hans Eysenck and Rudolph Grossarth-Maticek conducted studies on personality and stress coping. They concluded that this information can be very predictive of cancer and coronary heart disease.

How can so many different illnesses be related to stress?

The stress response causes the hypothalamus of the brain to trigger the adrenal glands to produce more "stress hormones," including adrenaline and cortisol. Adrenaline increases heart rate, elevates blood pressure, and increases energy supply. Cortisol increases the amount of sugar in the bloodstream, increases the brain's use of sugar, and makes substances that are used to repair body tissues more available. Cortisol also decreases certain vital functions, like immune system, digestive system, reproductive system, and growth functions. It does this to maximize fight-or-flight requirements during a threatening situation. The problem is that when the body interprets non-life-threatening stressors in the same way as life-threatening ones, it has the same type of reaction. The reaction can continue for much longer periods of time than intended, thus causing damage. Long-lasting stress connected to conditions that a person may believe they have little control over, like loss of a loved one, financial situation, being alone, caring for a severely ill child or parent over a long period of time, or a bad marriage, can actually weaken the immune system. The body has fewer defenses against things like viruses that cause colds, flu, cancer, herpes, and AIDS.

Stress can also affect the production of other hormones, other chemicals, prostaglandins (a class of unsaturated fatty acids that are involved in the contraction of smooth muscle, the control of inflammation and body temperature, and many other physiological functions), important enzymes (substances that boost chemical reactions in the body), and metabolic processes (processes in the body that produce energy). The stress reaction also has various effects on the digestive system and many organs, including the skin.

There are reasons why people have stomachaches, indigestion, heartburn, constipation, various pains, and skin problems at times when they are under stress. Damage is being done by the body's almost constant reaction to stress.

Stress can cause sleep problems. When you are preoccupied with problems and your nervous system is overexcited, it can be difficult to fall asleep or stay asleep.

Millions of Americans have difficulty sleeping. About 30 percent of American adults have insomnia, according to the American Academy of Sleep Medicine. These sleep problems lead to many problems. Dr. Dimitri Markov of the Jefferson Sleep Disorders Center in Philadelphia said insomnia can cause car accidents, depression, anxiety disorders, and weight problems. It can also play a role in heart disease and problems with pregnancy.

Dr. Eberto Pineiro, a neurologist at Watson Clinic, in Lakeland, Florida, thinks that an increase in sleeping problems might be caused by anxiety or depression.

If the sleep problems are not caused by bad bedtime habits, like reading or watching TV in bed, then they may be associated with depression or anxiety. In situations like this, some doctors say that medicines like Ambien or Lunesta might not even work. In these cases the depression or anxiety would need to be addressed in order for their sleep to improve.

Sometimes people who have trouble falling asleep automatically worry that they won't be able to fall asleep. They worry about not being able to sleep. As soon as it is time to go to bed, they start to think about not being able to sleep, and they usually do have trouble sleeping.

People who tend to dwell on problems or worry are more likely to have sleep problems.

Stress and Headaches, Neck, and Back Pain

People tend to tense or contract their muscles as a reaction to stress. This goes back to the fight-or-flight response that prepares the body for necessary action. The muscles contract so that you can react physically to a threatening situation. When there is no physical reaction required, the increased muscle contraction can be harmful rather than helpful. Normally after a threat or perceived threat has passed, the body should go back to a neutral, balanced state. The muscles should return to a relaxed state, waiting for the next time they are called upon before they contract again. When a person is constantly exposed to stress without the skills to deal with it properly, the body does not go back to that neutral state. The muscles remain partially contracted more than they should be. When this occurs for a long enough period of time, the result may be symptoms including headaches, neck pain, and back pain.

I worked as the biofeedback therapist in a pain management office for about eight years. I saw clients who were the victims of either motor vehicle or work accidents. Some of the most common complaints they had were headaches, neck pain, and back pain. I worked under the supervision of a licensed psychologist or psychiatrist. The medical doctor often prescribed muscle relaxant medication for the neck and back pain symptoms. I was not trained in medicine, but common sense told me that the medication was reducing the pain symptom because it was relaxing the muscles.

This must mean that the excess tension in the muscles was contributing to the pain. Many of the patients taking the muscle relaxant medication complained that they felt very lethargic. They felt like just staying in bed and sleeping or lying on the couch and watching TV all day. Their pain symptoms were reduced, but they couldn't really function.

The problem with a muscle relaxant is that it is not selective. It does not find the "problem muscle" that is too tense and relax only that one. It acts globally and relaxes all of the muscles, even the ones that were already relaxed. I used this information to explain how biofeedback could help them. EMG biofeedback shows the person how tense their muscles are. The person is able to learn to identify which muscle is too tense and to voluntarily relax that specific muscle. Relaxing the tense muscle usually reduces the pain in that area. This leaves the person still feeling alert and energetic rather than lethargic. He or she is better able to function because he or she has less pain without the side effect of feeling lethargic.

Chronic Stress and Disease

Even in our modern world, there are still times when the stress response is useful. When there is physical danger, or during sports activities that call for quick, rigorous muscle activity, the changes that happen in the body as a result of the stress response are useful and necessary, but only for a relatively short amount of time. Chronic stress is when stressors come one after another without a break or time for recovery. Things like reorganizations, downsizing, pay cuts, and layoffs at work, difficult divorces, and problems in a relationship or dealing with a long-term or serious sickness cause chronic stress reactions. Chronic stress can also come when smaller stressors add up and you do not recover from or deal properly with any of them. The body continues the stress response as long as the mind believes there is a threat. The longer the stress response occurs, the higher chance there is for the body to develop stress-related illness.

Research on the relationship between stress and disease has been going on for over fifty years. This research has shown that people are affected differently by ongoing stress reactions. Some of the systems of the body that are affected are skeletal, muscular, cardiovascular (involving the heart and/or blood vessels), and gastrointestinal (relating to the stomach and/or intestines).

Chronic stress causes muscle tension and fatigue for some people and hypertension, migraine headaches, ulcers, or chronic diarrhea in others.

Almost every system of the body can be damaged by stress. When stress affects the reproduction system, it can cause an interruption of normal menstruation and ovulation in women, impotency (erectile dysfunction) in men, and loss of libido (sexual desire) in both sexes.

When stress affects the lungs, symptoms of asthma, bronchitis (swelling of the mucous membranes of the bronchial tubes in the lungs), and other respiratory problems worsen.

Chronic stress response can also cause a decrease in insulin. This can contribute to the onset of diabetes in adults. Stress can slow down the repair of damaged tissue. This can lead to loss of calcium in the bones and osteoporosis (weakening and slowness to heal of bones) and makes it easier for bones to break. Stress slows down the immune and inflammatory systems, which makes you more susceptible to cold and flu and can make some diseases like cancer and AIDS worse. Long-lasting stress response can also make arthritis, chronic pain, and diabetes worse. Constant release and waste of norepinephrine (noradrenaline, a stress hormone that constricts blood vessels and causes increases in heart rate and blood pressure) during chronic stress can lead to depression.

The relationship between chronic stress, disease, and aging is also being researched. In our time some of the problems that go along with aging include cardiovascular disease, cancer, arthritis, respiratory problems like asthma and emphysema, and depression. Many of these problems appear to be sensitive to stress. Researchers are trying to figure out how stress speeds up the aging process and how this can be reversed or at least slowed down.

Cardiovascular diseases kill about one million Americans every year. This number amounts to about 50 percent of all deaths. Cancer causes about 25 percent of all deaths. One American dies of a cardiovascular disease every thirty-four seconds. One-fourth of all Americans have some sort of heart disease. Approximately 1,200,000 people have heart attacks in America. 500,000 of those people die. About 500,000 people have strokes. Sixty million have hypertension. Stress is not the only contributing factor in any of these conditions, but it is a contributing factor in all of them. Reducing stress could have a positive effect on these statistics.

Stress and the Immune System

Chronic stress has been called America's number one health problem by a few people, but the medical field as a system has not treated it as such. Symptoms are treated more often than sources. Stress should not be taken lightly. It can have tremendous effects on your immune system and the general state of your health.

Problems at work tend to be one of the top sources of stress for adults. There are also varied other sources, including crime, violence, peer pressure, substance abuse, family problems, social isolation, loneliness, and changes in religious values. These things can create problems for adults, children, teenagers, and the elderly.

Stress does not just mean worry. Many things that you might not think of that are related to stress can affect your body. Any change can be stressful. The stressful changes can be emotional, environmental, sickness, hormonal, or even working too hard. Sometimes even positive occasions, like getting a promotion on your job or taking a family vacation, can be stressful. The accumulated effects of these events can slowly weaken your health before you know it. Some of the signs that you are suffering from chronic stress are changes in your sleep patterns, feeling fatigued, anxiety, less enjoyment of life, and various aches and pains.

Short-term or long-term stress can have a negative effect on your immune system. Have you ever noticed that when you are under stress you are more likely to catch a cold or get the flu? Why? Your immune system is weakened by stress. According to professor of neurology and neurosurgery at Stanford University and author of *Why Zebras Don't Get Ulcers* Robert Sapolsky, when the body is responding to stress, normal functions like immune function are interrupted. Since the immune function is interrupted during stress, it is not doing the job it normally would do. This leaves the body more vulnerable to all types of illnesses and disease.

Chronic stress has a negative effect on stress partly because it affects the immune system. People who are under chronic stress have higher than normal levels of interleukin-6 (IL-6), an immune system protein that causes inflammation and has been associated with heart disease, diabetes, osteoporosis, rheumatoid arthritis, severe infections, and some cancers.

Stress seems to increase levels of IL-6, which in turn speeds up several age-related diseases. Stress can also weaken a person's immune response, leaving them more open to infection. Stress can also lead people to eat too much and not get enough sleep and/or exercise. All of these habits can create additional health problems.

Psychoneuroimmunology scientists (who study the effects of stress on the immune system) have discovered changes in the normal function of immune cells in animals during times of stress.

According to David Holland, MD, the medical communications director at Mediatrition:

> Excess physical stress also changes our immune cells. Increased upper respiratory tract infections occur in athletes who train too much. These athletes tend to have compromised immune function.

> Our bodies become vulnerable to invasion by germs like fungi, viruses and bacteria when our immune system is not working properly.

There is some scientific evidence that certain foods like garlic can help to prevent immune suppression caused by psychological stress.

As a rule people cannot avoid stress because it is all around us. We have to deal with it. The best we can do is to reduce our exposure to stress and realize the importance of dealing with stress before it has a negative effect on our health. Stress seems to impair the immune system. This allows infections that would normally be stopped by the immune system to cause damage to the body.

Most diseases are at least partially caused by infection. One example of this is autoimmune diseases like rheumatoid arthritis, which is partly a result of things like stress overload. Mild cases of rheumatoid arthritis can be improved through stress management techniques.

It is important to realize that stress can be a good thing. It increases your adrenaline and gives your body a boost to get things done. You need to be aware of your stress level and regulate it if stress starts to take over. Any stress that continues for too long without a break would tend to become a problem.

Stress and Obesity

Two out of three adults are overweight or obese, and the problem seems to be getting worse.

Stress can contribute to weight gain and obesity.

Excess weight can come as a result of stress reaction. Unmanaged stress can affect your appetite and weight. Your stress hormones are produced and sent into your bloodstream at a much higher rate than necessary.

As mentioned earlier cortisol is the adrenal stress hormone (chemical) that is released by the brain in response to stress. It is intended to help the body get ready for a physical response to a physical threat. I mention it again because cortisol stimulates an increase in appetite. If you are under stress regularly, the increased cortisol can push you to eat more, which has the result of increasing your weight.

The stress hormone levels in your bloodstream increase when you are affected by stress. The hormone causes fat cells to release fuel for what it thinks will be a fight-or-flight reaction. Your brain wrongly acts as though you are in a serious physical situation, so it restocks the body. These stressful situations do not require that we fight or run. Physical activity would use the fat as fuel. There is usually nothing physical to do.

When everyday stress occurs, we tend to suppress our natural response, which is driven by hormones. We usually just wait for the problem to pass. The problem is that the hormones are not suppressed. The hormones are still produced. But their effects are not needed. In these situations they are actually harmful to the body. The body then needs to repair itself, but it doesn't get the time to recover before something else happens to start the cycle again.

Cortisol is one of the main hormones released when we are under stress. It is intended to protect us from the source of the stress. High levels of cortisol in the body decrease protein in most body cells. They also make you want to eat and cause the body to store fat.

High levels of cortisol have also been connected to high blood sugar, rapid hair and bone loss, excess immune cell loss, and increased risk of infections. Appearing calm and collected on the outside while internally reacting to a high level of ongoing stress can help make us become obese.

There is scientific evidence that shows that when high stress hormone levels continue over a long period of time, many problems can result, including difficulty maintaining weight, reduced ability to feel relaxed, increased sugar or carbohydrate cravings, fatigue, a negative outlook, moodiness, increased PMS symptoms, and increased appetite. Elevated cortisol levels have been associated with a many negative health effects, like increased appetite, weight gain, diabetes, depression, and even heart disease and cancer. You can literally worry yourself sick!

It is normal for the stress hormone to be produced by your body in response to stressful events. This should be a relatively infrequent event that is necessary when responding to emergency situations. When cortisol is released too often in response to normal, daily stresses of our busy lives, it can have extremely negative health consequences.

In its role of preparing the body for action, the stress hormone increases blood pressure and heart rate, prepares stored fat, breaks down muscle and bone, suppresses the immune system, increases the appetite, and decreases sensitivity to insulin, which causes more fat to be stored. Usually the hormone does its job and then stops being produced. This allows your system to return to normal. But when you are under constant stress, your body reacts as though you are constantly in danger, so it continues to produce the stress hormones, and the levels remain higher than normal.

Psychological Factors

Because many people eat when they're stressed, bored, or angry, these problems can lead to weight gain. After a while the connection between emotions and food can become almost automatic and difficult to control.

Depression and stress are two of the top causes of obesity and eating disorders. Obesity can often be traced to behavioral or psychological problems. This does not always mean that a person is just weak or lacks willpower. It can be a sign of a mental disorder that is as serious as any physical problem that requires professional treatment.

Some medications can also cause obesity. Antidepressants and other medications that are used for the treatment of stress, anxiety, and depression can also cause weight gain as a side effect.

We are not forced to eat more than our bodies need. We don't have to be. Why is it that we seem to continue to be driven by hunger even when we have had enough food? This is sometimes called comfort eating. During the past twenty or more years, there has been a dramatic increase in the amount of food people are eating. Along with that increase, chronic disease diagnoses have also increased. During the same time, at a similar rate, the amount of stress in our society and on each of us individually has also increased.

Most people think about stress related to emotional states. There are many other things that can cause stress and negative health effects in our systems. Some of these other stress sources are not getting enough sleep or rest, too much work or exercise, poor nutrition, infections, allergies, injuries or trauma, dental or surgical procedures, or reproductive functions like pregnancy or menopause. The body adapts to survive.

It needs to have certain nutrition available for the kidney's adrenal glands to produce the correct hormones. When the body correctly or falsely detects that the nutrients are not available, hunger for foods that can cause unhealthy weight gain can result

According to MIT Professor Judith Wurtman, PhD, and others, a chemical messenger or neurotransmitter known as serotonin works to produce the desire for complex carbohydrates and sugars, which are two of the main nutritional substances that cause weight gain.

Serotonin is one of the neurotransmitters that are produced by our bodies to make us feel good. When we are under stress, we do not get enough of these substances, and we feel the need to do something that leads to the increase of serotonin so that we can feel good. Eating lots of carbohydrate and fat-rich foods, also known as "comfort foods," like cookies, ice cream, cakes, etc., greatly increases these neurotransmitters. Other addictions to substances like nicotine, alcohol, and drugs have the same goal of self-soothing by increase of serotonin, but these activities are nowhere near as socially acceptable and as easily available as eating too much food. It is totally legal, and it is offered to us constantly. We can overeat almost anywhere, anytime, alone or with company. It should not be surprising that overeating is such a prevalent problem.

Another contributing factor to overeating under stress is the dramatic increase in our body's demand for certain nutrients, including protein; vitamins A, C, and E; unsaturated fatty acids; cholesterol; and minerals. Unless the stress response pattern is interrupted or you supply your body with the nutrients it needs and craves, you will feel the need to overeat in order to satisfy the body's demands for nutrients.

When we eat comfort foods, we usually feel calmer for a while. When the serotonin level drops again, we start to feel burnt out again and feel the need to eat again. This type of behavior is sometimes called self-medication.

Over a long period of time, the effect of this behavior, besides obesity and an increase in chronic diseases, is that our nervous systems become overstimulated. When our nervous systems are overloaded, some of the symptoms we can develop are anxiety, exhaustion, depression, overeating, and insomnia.

This is why low-carbohydrate diets are helpful and effective for many people. One of the problems with low-carb diets being effective long-term is that if the stress response continues, a person may not be able to continue to resist the cravings of the body for carbohydrates to relieve the stress by increasing serotonin. If instead the stress response is reduced, then the need and desire for extra carbs and other nutrients will be reduced. This should lead to a reduction in overeating and a reduction in weight gain.

Most gym memberships are used for the first four to six weeks after signing up, and then use decreases dramatically. Gyms count on this when planning their marketing numbers. In the same way, diet plans and weight loss programs realize that more than 90 percent of their customers will continue to have weight problems even with the help of the program.

We live in a very competitive culture. One individual or group is against another individual or group. This kind of isolation causes a less obvious and almost continuous stress. This can lead to the exhaustion and the conditions that can contribute to overeating.

If you have a calm, smoothly operating nervous system, which is the life of the body, you don't need the latest diet craze or vitamin, drug, or surgery as much to treat obesity or other health problems.

Chapter 12

Stress and Accidents

Stress and driving = an accident waiting to happen. A man and his wife have an argument. He leaves the house, still upset. He gets into the car, forgets to put on his seat belt, and takes off. He drives faster than usual, changes lanes more abruptly and without signaling, races to beat the yellow light, speeds off as soon as the light turns green, forgetting that someone else at the intersection might be trying to beat the yellow light, just like he is doing. While driving on the highway, he tailgates and flashes his lights behind other cars even though they are going faster than the speed limit. One of the other drivers decides to pull into the other lane and curse him out as he passes them. He decides to pass and cut in front of them. Once in front he hits the brakes. You can imagine the possible results. People could get hurt or killed. Vehicles could be damaged. For what? Because of unmanaged stress—too short a fuse. Most accidents could probably be avoided. This type definitely could be.

It would be much better to take a five-minute walk first to burn up some of the extra physical energy. After this he could get in the car and take a few deep breaths before putting on his seat belt and driving off. This simple change could produce a totally different result. Much of the edge would likely be greatly reduced. He would probably not be nearly as on edge and aggressive.

Work Accidents

Decreased efficiency and chronic fatigue are often the results of stress. Our senses can be negatively affected by chronic stress. The overstimulation of stress can cause our senses to become less sensitive. Under stress a person may become less focused on details, less aware of what is happening around him or her, and may ignore many important sensations and experiences. This is when we are more likely to make mistakes. This state of carelessness can lead to serious farm accidents. In fact, it has been found that besides mining, farming has one of the highest rates of accidents of any type of work. Farmers become more accident-prone when they are under stress. The accident rates in high- and low-stress jobs are alarming. It isn't just that some jobs are more dangerous; highly stressed people have more accidents when they are not on the job too (Lehmann 1974).

Think of all of the dangerous jobs that people perform. Some examples are construction, factory work, cutting wood or metal, operating heavy equipment like forklifts and cranes, driving, surgery, dispensing medication. A person has to stay focused on what he or she is doing. But even when a person is focused, sometimes accidents happen. Imagine how easily an accident can happen when a person is stressed out.

Stress management training for employees would likely decrease accidents in the workplace.

Chapter 13

Stress and Education

Stress can have a negative effect in educational settings just as it can in the workplace. Students who are under stress do not perform at their potential. A student may know the information, but if he or she is under stress, his or her mind may go blank when it is time to perform on a test. He or she might also be distracted when lessons are taught so that the information is not absorbed in the first place. Teachers who are under stress cannot give the students their best either.

I had the opportunity to return to Ossining High School (I graduated from OHS with the class of 1984) along with Elizabeth Stroebel, PhD, creator of the Kiddie-QR Program (a stress management program created specifically for children) to teach a course on biofeedback and stress management for students for a group of educators from the school district.

The goal of the course was to help educators become more aware of how much of a problem stress can be in the school environment, both for students and staff. I also showed them how biofeedback and simple relaxation techniques could be used to help manage stress. The group was made up of regular classroom teachers, special education teachers, speech therapists, guidance counselors, and a music teacher.

The participants were very enthusiastic about the information we shared with them. Here are some of the questions that I asked the group, along with answers we came up with:

Question: What are some of the sources of stress for students?

Answer: Exams, problems at home, work, bullies, added responsibility of having to help support the family financially, keeping up with fashion, peer pressure, relationship problems with teachers, learning disabilities, and pressure to get into a good college

Question: What are some signs that school staff can notice in students that indicate possible reaction to stress?

Answer: Hunched or raised shoulders, tapping of foot or pencil, sad appearance or affect, head down, withdrawn, demonstrations of anger, aggression, clenched jaw or fist, lack of focus, fatigue, and rapid, shallow breathing

Question: What are some of the negative effects stress can have in the school setting?

Answer: Visits to the nurse's office due to headaches and stomachaches, arguments, physical fights, disruption in class, inattention in class, lack of focus, test anxiety, decreased cognitive abilities, poor performance, decreased participation, student/teacher relationship problems

Question: What is currently being done to deal with stress in the school setting?

Answer: Mentoring programs and counselors are available for students to talk to; yoga is now offered as an alternative to standard gym; a crisis team is in place to deal with major problems that come up, like the death of a student or other major school or community tragedy

Question: What else can be done to help reduce stress in the school environment?

Answer: Offer a course on stress management and biofeedback as part of staff development. One participant suggested that this would help teachers become more aware of what causes stress, signs of stress, and how to better help students reduce stress, as well as how not to add to the stress of students. Other suggestions included introducing students to biofeedback so they could actually see their stress levels and learn how to reduce them, creating a more relaxing atmosphere, improving relationships between teachers and students, offering stress management training to parents and making them aware of biofeedback, setting up biofeedback in the "time out" room, and creating a relaxing space that students could retreat to if needed.

Question: What are some of the challenges/roadblocks in implementing biofeedback/stress management programs in schools?

Answer: Money, bureaucracy, attitudes/perceptions, willingness to participate, space, language barriers

Question: How could these challenges/roadblocks be resolved?

Answer: Apply for grants; provide students, parents, administrators, and community with information and demonstration of how stress management and biofeedback works; accumulate data from research showing a strong positive correlation between stress reduction and management and student achievement; offer workshops for district policy makers to demonstrate the effectiveness of reducing stress on student performance and behavior

This was a very enjoyable and enlightening experience for me. The participants said that they learned a lot about stress, stress management, and biofeedback. I learned a lot about stress in the school setting. It was very fulfilling to return to my old school and be able to share some of what I have learned since my graduation back in 1984. My hope is that I will be able to help incorporate stress management and biofeedback into this school district to help the students and staff improve their performance and lives.

Chapter 14

Solutions

What can you do about stress?

Some ways of dealing with stress are ineffective or not my first choice for some other reason.

Doctors have traditionally treated the symptoms that arise from stress reactions. They prescribe drugs/medications to reduce pain, help you fall asleep and stay asleep, keep you awake, help you relax, and help with acid indigestion and nervous stomach/bowels. Some people use eating, drinking alcohol, smoking, and drugs like marijuana to help deal with the symptoms related to stress reactions. These methods are very limited in their effectiveness. Most of them also carry with them unwanted side effects.

Here are two examples of the medications that are used to treat stress symptoms, as well as usage warnings and side effect warnings:

Alprazolam (Brand name: Xanax)

Benzodiazepine anxiolytic

Anxiety disorders: Adults

Panic disorders

This drug comes with warnings against using it for pregnant women, mothers who are nursing, patients under eighteen years old, psychotic or depressed patients, older people, and patients with kidney or liver problems. There is also a warning against prescribing it for people who may have abused drugs or alcohol.

Some of the side effects listed are drowsiness, dizziness, coordination problems, hostility, irritability, and hallucinations.

Isn't this terrible? A drug that is supposed to help with anxiety and panic can actually make you hostile and irritable.

There are also warnings about interactions with other drugs, like antifungal medications and certain antibiotics. Taking alprazolam (Xanax) while drinking alcohol or other substances that depress the central nervous system can be a problem too. It is recommended that you don't drive while using the drug because of dizziness and drowsiness.

Taking these drugs is not the simple quick fix it seems to be on the television commercials. All of the negative effects and warnings are said so fast and listed in such fine print that it is obvious that we are not supposed to see or hear them. They are just there to cover a legal obligation and help prevent lawsuits.

A person taking this drug may not be able to perform some of his or her normal activities because it decreases mental alertness, judgment, and physical coordination. Activities like driving or using potentially dangerous machinery should be avoided, especially when the person first starts taking it and until he or she has adjusted to side effects.

It has not been determined to be safe to use during pregnancy. Some studies have shown the possibility of an increased risk of birth defects associated with the use of the benzodiazepines during the first trimester of pregnancy.

Rat studies have shown that alprazolam and its traces are passed through the milk. Because of this mothers should not nurse their babies while taking this drug.

Precautions

Alprazolam can cause a drop in blood pressure in older patients that could lead to heart problems. It could also cause them to be overly sedated, and it could have negative effects on their brain functions.

There is a risk of dependency for people who are prone to substance abuse. They may suffer withdrawal symptoms, including irritability, nervousness, insomnia, shaking, vomiting, mental impairment, diarrhea, and stomach cramps, if they stop taking the drug.

Some people who have emotional problems may have suicidal feelings if they take this drug, especially if they are depressed.

If alprazolam is used over a long period of time, it is recommended that the patient's blood and liver function be tested regularly. This would lead me to believe that it could be doing damage to the blood and liver; otherwise why test them?

There are many possible undesirable side effects. The most commonly reported are sleepiness, decreased coordination, dizziness, hostile behavior, irritability, excitability and hallucinations.

Clomipramine (Brand name: Anafranil)

Pharmacology

Antidepressant/Antiobsessional

Clomipramine helps with symptoms of depression and obsession.

It seems to have a mild calming effect, which can help decrease the anxiety that often comes with depression.

Clomipramine causes desynchronization of EEG (electroencephalograph, electrical activity) in the brain. It causes a persistent increase in the frequency of shifts into stage I sleep and produces substantial reduction of rapid eye movement sleep (REM) with partial recovery within three to four weeks and a rebound after drug withdrawal that appears to last approximately the same time. In normal people this type of drug has a relaxing effect, but it can cause difficulty in focused thinking.

Serious problems can occur if clomipramine is given with or within two weeks of treatment with a MAO inhibitor (a type of drug used to treat depression or Parkinson's disease). Hypersensitivity, hyperactivity, hyperpyrexia (high fever), spasticity, severe convulsions, and coma have been reported. Some patients that have received this combination have even died.

It can be dangerous to give clomipramine to people with certain heart problems, existing liver or kidney damage, history of abnormal blood conditions, or glaucoma.

A potential negative side effect is an irregular heartbeat. There have been a few unexpected deaths reported in patients with cardiovascular problems. Heart attack and stroke have also been reported connected with this type of drug.

This drug has not been proven to be safe for pregnant women. Some babies born to women on clomipramine-type drugs have suffered from withdrawal symptoms, including tremors, convulsions, and breathing problems. It also passes into breast milk, so if a mother did take the drug she wouldn't be able to breast-feed.

Precautions

There is an increased risk of suicide for depressed people taking clomipramine. There is also a risk of overdose, so it is prescribed in very small quantities.

Clomipramine causes sedation, so patients have to be warned against doing things that call for mental alertness, judgment, and physical coordination.

Other potential problems include liver damage, bone marrow depression, allergic skin reaction, fever, flu, hyperthermia, withdrawal symptoms including dizziness, nausea, vomiting, headache, a general sense of depression, unease, and discomfort, sleep disturbance, hyperthermia and irritability, and tooth decay.

Negative effects:

Stomach problems, dry mouth, constipation, nausea, dyspepsia, and anorexia; nervous system complaints, including drowsiness, tremor, dizziness, nervousness and muscle spasm; complaints including changed libido, problems with ejaculation, impotence and urination disorder; and other miscellaneous complaints, including fatigue, sweating, increased appetite, weight gain, and changes in sight.

There are many more medications that are used for treating stress disorders, but it is not the goal of this book to detail them. Suffice it to say that medication is one way to deal with stress, but it is a very imperfect and usually not a permanent solution. There are many side effects, and because it is not a permanent fix, a person may need to continue using the drug for a long time, which can be expensive financially and in the various other ways listed above.

Eating to Relieve Stress

Eating too much can lead to obesity, hypertension, heart disease, diabetes, and joint problems.

Drinking Alcohol to Relieve Stress

Drinking too much alcohol can lead to liver disease, and it has a depressive effect on the brain; it can also change the structure and function of the kidneys. Excessive alcohol consumption can reduce the ability of the kidneys to regulate the amount and composition of fluids and electrolytes in the body.

Smoking to Relieve Stress

Smoking can lead to lung cancer, cardiovascular disease, emphysema, negative effects of brain function and tissue, erectile dysfunction, sinus problems, and decreased immune function.

Use of Illegal Drugs to Relieve Stress

Use of illegal drugs like marijuana can lead to memory problems, sleepiness, anxiety, paranoia, nausea, headaches, reduced brain blood flow, changes in reproductive organs, and of course arrest since it is illegal.

Other Common Diversions to Relieve Stress:

Some people use diversions like TV, movies, hobbies, video games, or sports to keep their minds off of the sources or effects of stress. Although these diversions seem harmless, too much of any of these can lead to a decrease in productivity and time spent with family, which can lead to relationship problems. Some people start withdrawing from the world and staying home to avoid stressors, but who wants to do that? This can lead to social isolation, which itself is stressful, and depression. Even if you don't leave your home, some stress will still find you there. There's no hiding place.

Counseling

A mental health counselor, psychotherapist, psychologist, or other qualified therapist can provide solid advice and be someone to hear you talk about your stress. They are trained to provide various techniques and information that will help you to manage your stress.

Biofeedback

Biofeedback is a process in which we use electronic instruments to measure the responses of the body to stress. We can measure brain wave activity, muscle tension, skin temperature, skin conductance (sweat activity), heart rate, and respiration. The signals are measured using sensors connected to an instrument. The instrument shows the person who is connected to it what the levels are and how they are changing in response to stress or relaxation. We use biofeedback instruments to teach people how they are reacting negatively to stress, and then we help them learn how to relax using the instruments as a guide.

Biofeedback is a tool like a mirror that helps you to see if there is something you need to change, what direction you need to change it in, and how much progress you are making in meeting your goal of change. Two examples are bathroom scales and lane markings on the highway. A bathroom scale allows you to see if the things you are doing are causing you to gain or lose weight. Changes that you make in diet, exercise, and so on will be reflected in what you see when you get on the scale. When you are driving on the highway, the lane markings tell you if you need to make adjustments in your steering to the left or right.

Here is an example of how a biofeedback instrument can show what happens when a person reacts negatively to repeated stressors without complete recovery. These screens are from the Biograph Infiniti Biofeedback Software and recorded using the Biograph Infiniti hardware, both made by Thought Technology Ltd. of Montreal, Canada.

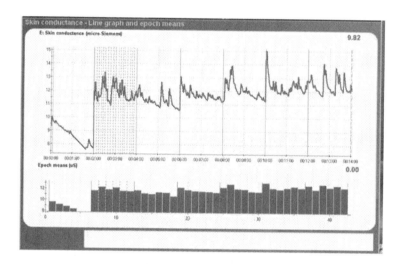

Skin conductance is one of the signals we can measure that shows responses to stress. It is based on sweat activity. The units of measure are called microsiemens. Sensors are placed on the palm side of two fingers. The conductance reading changes based on the amount of sweat on the skin. Less sweat gives a lower reading. More sweat is produced during a stress response, which causes a higher reading.

The above image expresses graphically a case where repeated stress responses without recovery cause a person's skin conductance (sweat gland activity) to increase to a much higher level than baseline. When the level first increased from 7.76 microsiemens to 13.23 microsiemens, the person could have practiced a relaxation exercise that might have returned the level to 7.76. Instead, another stressor occurred that caused the level to increase further. This was repeated until the level ended up at 15.05, 7.29 microsiemens higher than where it started. This is a 94 percent increase. At this level it is much more difficult to recover to where you started. When you become just a little upset, it is easier to calm down. When you become extremely upset, it is much more difficult to calm down. This is similar to what happens in a panic attack. The anxiety level passes the point where a person still has the ability to return to feeling normal. He or she gets to the point where he or she needs help to calm down.

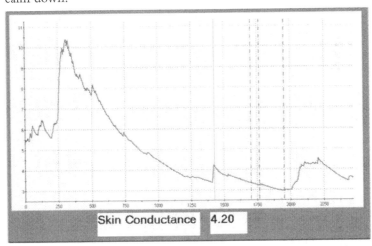

The above graph shows an increase in skin conductance from about 5.5 microsiemens to about 10.3 microsiemens. This is followed by a recovery where the level decreases to 3.5, which is even lower than where it started. Now, when the next stressor causes an increase, it only brings it up to 4.2. If there had not been a recovery, the level would be 11.1. After this increase comes another recovery, which brings the level down to 3, even lower than before. The next reaction brings the level to 4.3. Without the two recovery periods, the level would have reached 12.3. This is a huge difference and could mean the difference between reaching the "boiling point,"

the "straw that broke the camel's back," the "breaking point," the point where "I just can't take any more," or the point where "I lost it."

Here is another example of the difference between managing stress and stress getting out of control. A person puts a pot of water on the stove. He turns the fire off every two minutes and drops in a few ice cubes before turning the fire back on. He continues this for thirty minutes. Another person puts a pot of water on the fire and leaves the fire on for thirty minutes straight. Which one will reach boiling first? The answer is obvious.

You can increase your ability to deal with distress.

According to Herbert Benson, an expert in the area of relaxation, you can use your mind to change your physiology for the better. This can improve your health and possibly the need for certain medications. Benson came up with the phrase "the relaxation response."

The opposite of the stress response is the relaxation response. It is activated by the same mechanism. When you decide that the situation is not dangerous anymore, your brain stops sending the emergency signals to the brain stem, and the brain stem stops sending panic messages to the nervous system. It takes about three minutes after the danger signals stop for the fight-or-flight response to wear out. The metabolism, heart rate, breath rate, muscle tension, and blood pressure then return to their pre-event levels.

There are some things that you can do nutritionally to help reduce the effects of chronically elevated stress hormones. Eating fresh, natural whole foods is helpful. Reducing your intake of processed and artificial foods also helps. You should also avoid caffeine and sugar.

Essential Oils

Essential oils are distilled from plants. They are natural and don't have the side effects that are common from many medications. Many cultures have historically used plants as medicine. Essential oils have also been used in many ancient religions for various purposes. Unlike pharmaceutical medications, essential oils don't tend to have negative side effects. Instead they usually have multiple positive side benefits.

Lavender: Calms the mind and body, reduces nervous tension, encourages inner peace. A

1998 study showed changes in brain wave patterns of people who inhaled lavender essential oil.

Another study concluded "the lavender oil aroma significantly decreased mean scores for anxiety."

Cedarwood: A key stress-relieving oil because it stimulates the limbic region of the brain, specifically the pineal gland, which releases melatonin, which plays a role in establishing sleep cycles and can help bring stability and calm.

Frankincense: Frankincense oil is rich in sesquiterpene molecules, which stimulate many of the centers of the limbic system, including the hypothalamus, pineal and pituitary glands. 2008 research demonstrated lowered anxiety and antidepressant behavior in mice. The researchers extrapolated that the ancient practice of burning frankincense activated little-known ion channels in the brain and created a state of calm that relieved anxiety and depression.

Not all essential oils are the same. Some are pure, and some are cut or mixed with other oils, making them less effective. The type that I use is so pure that most can be taken internally. Contact me if you would like more information on acquiring pure essential oils.

E-mail: Harry@biofeedbackinternational.com

Some herbs that can help reduce stress are licorice root, passionflower, kava, and St. John's wort.

Yoga

According to a 2011 Psychology Today article, there is scientific research to prove that yoga reduces stress, pain, blood pressure, and depression.

Meditation

The Mayo Clinic staff says, "If stress has you anxious, tense, and worried, consider trying meditation. Spending even a few minutes in meditation can restore your calm and inner peace."

Stress Reduction exercises

Progressive muscle relaxation, autogenic relaxation training, diaphragmatic breathing, Quieting Reflex™, and Freeze Frame™ can all be helpful.

What happens when you relax?

Your immune system works better.

You feel more positive.

Your senses—hearing, sight, taste, smell, etc.—become more acute.

Chemicals called endorphins are produced by the brain. These chemicals can reduce the perception of pain, boost healing, and generally make you feel good.

There are many tools for managing stress, including biofeedback instruments that you can use at home, books, audio CDs, and videos at www.mindbodydevices.com

Consider developing a regular exercise program. Massage is also a very good method of reducing stress.

I recommend that you find a local stress management or biofeedback provider if you would like to receive professional help. This is usually a good idea at least at the beginning. After working with a professional, you can ask him or her for recommendations for continued home practice for maintenance.

Chapter 15

Conclusion

I hope that by now you are more aware of how serious the problem of stress is in our individual lives, in our communities, and in the world as a whole. Stress can touch so many parts of our lives. It affects our mood, health, happiness, finances, performance, and so much more. That's the bad news. The good news is that there are many things that we can do to manage and react to the stress that cannot be avoided. Stress is not something to just shrug off and say there is nothing to be done about it. Be aware of it. Avoid it when possible. Do the things that are in your power to minimize the negative effects of it when it can't be avoided. You will have a happier, healthier, and more productive life.

Contact Biofeedback Resources International and request a *free* stress card to practice stress reduction techniques anywhere you go. Just mention this book, and we will send you a free stress card.

Go to the websites listed below to order stress management tools, including books, audio and video material, biofeedback tools, and more.

Toll Free: 877-669-6463 or 914-762-4646

Web:　　　www.mindbodydevices.com

www.biofeedbackinternational.com

E-mail: info@biofeedbackinternational.com

Additional copies of this book can also be ordered from Biofeedback Resources International by calling 914-762-4646. Ask about quantity discounts if you would like copies for groups, associations, schools, teams, or companies.

To arrange to have Mr. Campbell speak for your group, association, school, team, or company, call 914-762-4646 or send an e-mail to Harry@biofeedbackinternational.com.

Other Helpful Websites

Northeast Regional Biofeedback Society: www.nrbs.org

Association for Applied Psychophysiology & Biofeedback (AAPB): www.aapb.org

The Biofeedback Certification International Alliance BCIA) www.bcia.org

The American Institute of Stress: www.stress.org

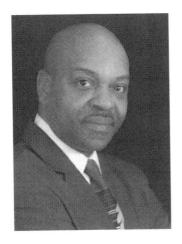

Harry L. Campbell Contact Information

Twitter @biofeedbackman.com

Facebook Personal: Harry L. Campbell

Facebook Corporate Fan Page: Biofeedback Resources International

LinkedIn: Harry L. Campbell

Podcast/Blog: BiofeedbackResources.Podbean.com

References

Sapolsky, R. *Why Zebras Don't Get Ulcers*

Stress, Portrait of a Killer DVD, National Geographic

Stress and Your Body, The Great Courses DVD series

Occup Environ Med. Nov 1998; 55(11): 729–734.

The Walker Survey of stress symptoms in farmers

Robert Karasek and Töres Theorell, Basic Books, 1990, *Healthy Work: Stress, Productivity, and the Reconstruction of Working Life*

Work Stress Statistics

The 2000 Integra Survey

Attitudes in the American Workplace VI poll, sponsored by the Marlin Company

Stranks and Dewis, *RoS Health and Safety Practice*, Pitman, 1986

McEwen, Bruce., S, N Engl J Med 1998; 338:171-179 January 15, 1998

Carlson, Scott, *The Chronicle of Higher Education* titled "The Net Generation Goes to College," October 7, 2005

Jenkins, Henry, "*Confronting the Challenges of Participatory Culture: Media Education for the 21st Century,*"

Boorstein, Sylvia, *Don't Just Do Something, Sit There: A Mindfulness Retreat*

Natural Law Party (www.natural-law.org/platform/crime.html)

USA TODAY. Nov 13, 1995,p 1A 20. Jones L: Gun advocates try to shoot...

Alcoholism Treatment Quarterly 11:89–117, 1994

Archives of General Psychiatry 49:429-435, 436–441, 1992; Life Sciences 33:2609–2614, 1983

Petersilia, J., "Crime and Punishment in California; Full Cells, Empty Pockets, and Questionable Benefits, "CPS Brief Berkley CA: California Policy Seminars May 1993.

Sapolsky, R., Stress, the Aging Brain, and the mechanisms of Neuron Death, Cambridge, MA: MIT Press, 1992

Journal of Clinical Psychology 45:957–974, 1989; Society of Neuroscience Abstracts 18:1541, 1992; Journal of Neural Transmission 39:257–267, 1976; Criminal justice and Behavior 5:3–20, 1978; Dissertation Abstracts International, 51:5048, 1991.

"The Root Causes of Crime" (CS&CPC Statement on the Root Causes of Crime, approved in 1996)

"Post-traumatic stress disorder is now the big problem in Sandy-stricken areas", The Daily News, May 23, 2013

Wolf, S. "The Scales of Libra: Social Factors That Influence Stress", The First International Congress on Stress, 1988

Sigerist, H. Civilization and Disease., 1944

Stacy, B., Cancer Stress and Death, 2013

Vilhjalmur, S. Cancer: Disease of Civilization

Time Magazine "Stress, the Epidemic of the Eighties, June 6, 1983,

Friedman, M and Rosenman, R., Type A Behavior and Your Heart," 1974,

Daniel Goleman, PhD, Emotional Intelligence, and Destructive Emotions

Alcohol's Impact on Kidney Function

Murray Eptein, M.D. Alcohol, Health & Research World Vol 21, No 1, 1997

About the Author

- Certified by Biofeedback Certification International Alliance (BCIA)

- Certified by B.C.I. (Biofeedback Consultants, Inc.)

- Bachelor of Professional Studies in Wellness and Health Care Technology from The State University of New York, Empire State College

- Board member of the Ossining Teacher's Staff Development Center for the Ossining Union Free School District

- President of Biofeedback Resources International Corp (formerly American Biotec Corporation) and has worked with the organization since 1984; Mr. Campbell purchased the business from Adam Crane, the previous owner, after working with the company for over twenty-two years

- Provided biofeedback for motor vehicle and workplace accident victims at a pain management clinic in the Bronx, New York, from 1988 to 2005

- Helped set up an EEG biofeedback program in the Yonkers public school system along with Mary Jo Sabo, PhD, of Biofeedback Consultants Inc. and Linda Vergara

- On staff at the Star Center for Psychotherapy & Well Being in Ossining, New York, 2000–2003

- On staff with Psychological & Biofeedback Services of Westchester 2012 – present

Mr. Campbell has trained hundreds of professionals in biofeedback and the use of biofeedback equipment for Health Training Seminars, the training division of Biofeedback Resources International Corp. He has also been hired to perform staff training in biofeedback and stress management at hospitals and clinics throughout the country, including Harlem Hospital, St. Vincent's Medical Center, Sloan-Kettering, Pace University, York College, Holy Name Hospital, VA Medical Center (the Bronx, New York), VA Medical Center (West Haven, Connecticut), Pope Air Force Base, Shaw Air Force Base (Charleston, South Carolina), Naval Brig, Charleston, SC, Groton, Connecticut Submarine Base, and the Naval Medical Center of Bethesda, Maryland., Boston Medical Center

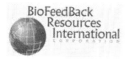

33935251R00062

Made in the USA
Middletown, DE
02 August 2016